Department of International Economic and Social Affairs

ST/ESA/SER.A/107

Population Studies No. 107

Step-by-Step Guide to the Estimation of Child Mortality

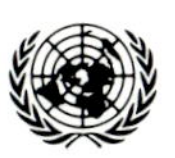

United Nations New York, 1990

ST/ESA/SER.A/107

PREFACE

In 1983 estimates of the levels and trends of infant mortality for all the countries of the world were first published by the Population Division of the Department of International Economic and Social Affairs of the United Nations Secretariat, with the support and encouragement of the United Nations Children's Fund (UNICEF) and the assistance of the World Health Organization (WHO) and the United Nations regional commissions (United Nations, 1983a). Since then, those estimates and projections have been updated twice by the United Nations (United Nations, 1986 and 1988). Recently, an additional indicator of child mortality—namely, mortality of children under the age of 5—was added (United Nations, 1988). Because of the lack of reliable vital-registration statistics in most developing countries, the available estimates are often obtained by the use of indirect estimation methods.

Aware of the possible problems in the interpretation and use of such methods, UNICEF, which has played an important role in disseminating information about levels and trends of mortality in childhood, requested the Population Division of the United Nations Secretariat to prepare the present guide to the estimation of child mortality in order to familiarize a wide audience with the estimation methods most commonly used and their strengths and limitations.

From a demographic perspective, the *Guide* is closely related to the series of Population Division manuals aimed at promoting widespread understanding and use of the estimation methods developed in the various population fields. Though the *Guide* is simpler and less comprehensive than other manuals covering similar topics, it does not sacrifice substance to simplification and thus provides a solid basis for understanding all the intricacies of the methods available. It is thus useful both for the demographer wishing to master those methods and for the non-demographer whose aim is to become familiar with their main traits.

To accompany the *Guide,* a program for microcomputers, named QFIVE, was prepared by the Population Division expressly to apply the Brass method as described here.* Special thanks are due to Kenneth Hill of Johns Hopkins University, who wrote a preliminary version of the *Guide.* It was later expanded by the Population Division, in order to make its contents more accessible to those who are not familiar with recent demographic techniques.

Acknowledgement is also due to UNICEF for providing part of the financial support that made the *Guide* possible.

---

*Inquiries concerning the QFIVE program should be directed to the Director, Population Division, United Nations, New York, New York 10017.

CONTENTS

		Page
PREFACE		iii
INTRODUCTION		1

Chapter

I.	INDICATORS OF MORTALITY IN CHILDHOOD	3
	Life tables	3
	Measurement of mortality in childhood	5
	Cohort versus period measures of mortality in childhood	6
	Model life tables	7
	Observed patterns of mortality in childhood and the model life tables	10
II.	DATA REQUIRED FOR THE BRASS METHOD	13
	Nature of the data required	13
	Children ever born and children dead	13
	Total female population of reproductive age	14
	Compilation of the data required	14
	The case of Bangladesh	14
III.	RATIONALE OF THE BRASS METHOD	22
	Allowing for the age pattern of child-bearing	22
	Derivation of the method	23
	Estimating time trends of mortality	23
	Limitations of the Brass method associated with its simplifying assumptions	23
IV.	TRUSSELL VERSION OF THE BRASS METHOD	25
	Computational procedure	25
	A detailed example	27
	Compilation of the data required	27
	Computational procedure	29
	Estimates of mortality in childhood by sex	32
V.	PALLONI-HELIGMAN VERSION OF THE BRASS METHOD	34
	Data required	34
	Computational procedure	34
	A detailed example	38
	Compilation of the data required	38
	Computational procedure	38
	Estimations of mortality in childhood by sex	45
VI.	INTERPRETATION AND USE OF THE ESTIMATES YIELDED BY THE BRASS METHOD	46
	Which version of the Brass method should one use?	46
	Use of information on the pattern of mortality in childhood to test the adequacy of mortality models	46
	What are the consequences of using the "wrong" model?	48
	Analysis of data from successive censuses or surveys	50
	Overall observations on the use of the Brass method	53
VII.	BRASS-MACRAE METHOD	56
	Nature of the basic data	56
	Derivation of the method and its rationale	57
	Limitations of the Brass-Macrae method	57
	Application of the Brass-Macrae method	57
	Data required	57
	Computational procedure	58
	A detailed example	58
	Comments on the results of the method	59

ANNEXES   *Page*

I.   Coale-Demeny model life table values for probabilities of dying between birth and exact age x, $q(x)$ 61

II.   United Nations model life table values for probabilities of dying between birth and exact age x, $q(x)$ 68

III.   Relationship between infant mortality, $q(1)$, and child mortality, $_4q_1$, in the Coale-Demeny mortality models 79

IV.   Relationship between infant mortality, $q(1)$, and child mortality, $_4q_1$, in the United Nations mortality models 80

NOTES 81

GLOSSARY 82

REFERENCES 83

TABLES

1.   Example of a life table 3

2.   Estimates of the probabilities of dying by ages 1 and 5, $q(1)$ and $q(5)$, by major region, 1950-1955, 1965-1970 and 1980-1985 6

3.   Correspondence between observed proportions of children dead by age group of mother and estimated probabilities of dying 23

4.   Coefficients for the estimation of child mortality multipliers, $k(i)$, Trussell version of the Brass method, using the Coale-Demeny mortality models 26

5.   Coefficients for the estimation of the time reference, $t(i)$, for values of $q(x)$, Trussell version of the Brass method, using the Coale-Demeny mortality models 27

6.   Calculation of the sex ratio at birth from data on children ever born, classified by sex, from the 1974 Bangladesh Retrospective Survey 29

7.   Application of the Trussell version of the Brass method to data on both sexes from the 1974 Bangladesh Retrospective Survey 30

8.   Application of the Trussell version of the Brass method to data on males from the 1974 Bangladesh Retrospective Survey 32

9.   Application of the Trussell version of the Brass method to data on females from the 1974 Bangladesh Retrospective Survey 32

10.   Coefficients for the estimation of child-mortality multiplers, $k(i)$, Palloni-Heligman version of the Brass method, using the United Nations mortality models 36

11.   Coefficients for the estimation of the time reference, $t(i)$, for values of $q(x)$, Palloni-Heligman version of the Brass method, using the United Nations mortality models 37

12.   Application of the Palloni-Heligman version of the Brass method to data on males from the 1974 Bangladesh Retrospective Survey 41

13.   Application of the Palloni-Heligman version of the Brass method to data on females from the 1974 Bangladesh Retrospective Survey 44

14.   Application of the Palloni-Heligman version of the Brass method to data on both sexes from the 1974 Bangladesh Retrospective Survey 45

15.   Comparison of estimated infant and under-five mortality in Bangladesh with the available mortality models 47

16.   Estimates of infant and under-five mortality in Bangladesh, obtained using the Coale-Demeny mortality models 48

17.   Estimates of infant and under-five mortality in Bangladesh, obtained using the United Nations mortality models 49

18.   Estimation of under-five mortality in Tunisia from data from successive censuses, using model West and the Trussell version of the Brass method 51

19.   Estimation of under-five mortality in Ecuador from data from several sources, using model West and the Trussell version of the Brass method 54

20.   Estimation of the probability of dying, $q(x)$, for Bamako, Mali, using the Brass-Macrae method 58

21.   Estimation of the probability of dying by age 2, $q(2)$, for Solomon Islands, using the Brass-Macrae method 59

FIGURES

1.   Typical shapes of the $1(x)$ and $_1q_x$ functions of a life table 4

2.   Relation between cohort and period measures shown by a Lexis diagram 7

vi

Page

3. Relationship between infant mortality, $q(1)$, and child mortality, ${}_4q_1$, in the Coale-Demeny mortality models 8
4. Relationship between infant mortality, $q(1)$, and child mortality, ${}_4q_1$, in the United Nations mortality models 9
5. Comparison of country-specific estimates of infant and child mortality with the Coale-Demeny mortality models 10
6. Comparison of country-specific estimates of infant and child mortality with the United Nations mortality models 11
7. Under-five mortality, $q(5)$, for both sexes in Bangladesh, estimated using model South and the Trussell version of the Brass method.................... 31
8. Under-five mortality, $q(5)$, for males and females in Bangladesh, estimated using model South and the Trussell version of the Brass method.................... 33
9. Under-five mortality, $q(5)$, for males in Bangladesh, estimated using the South Asian model and the Palloni-Heligman version of the Brass method.................... 43
10. Under-five mortality, $q(5)$, for males and females in Bangladesh, estimated using the South Asian model and the Palloni-Heligman version of the Brass method.................... 44
11. Comparison of the estimates of under-five mortality in Bangladesh, obtained using models South and South Asian.................... 47
12. Infant and under-five mortality for both sexes in Bangladesh, estimated using the four Coale-Demeny mortality models 50
13. Infant and under-five mortality for both sexes in Bangladesh, estimated using the five United Nations mortality models.................... 51
14. Range of variation of the possible estimates of infant and under-five mortality for both sexes in Bangladesh.................... 52
15. Under-five mortality for both sexes in Tunisia, estimated using model West and the Trussell version of the Brass method 53
16. Under-five mortality for both sexes in Ecuador, estimated using model West and the Trussell version of the Brass method.................... 54

DISPLAYS

1. Possible combinations for the compilation of the data on children ever born and children dead by age of mother required by the Brass method 15
2. Possible combinations for the compilation of the data on the total number of women of reproductive age required by the Brass method.................... 16
3. Tabulation of data on children ever born and children surviving as appearing in the report on the 1974 Bangladesh Retrospective Survey of Fertility and Mortality 17
4. Tabulation of the female population by age group and marital status as appearing in the report on the 1974 Bangladesh Retrospective Survey of Fertility and Mortality 18
5. First step in the compilation of data on children ever born and children dead for Bangladesh.................... 19
6. Second step in the compilation of data on children ever born and children dead for Bangladesh.................... 20
7. Compilation of data on the total number of women by age group for Bangladesh 21
8. Alternative compilation of data on the total number of women by age group for Bangladesh (data rejected in the application of the Brass method) 21
9. Worksheet for the compilation of data on births in a year by age group of mother for the Palloni-Heligman version of the Brass method.................... 35
10. Tabulation of data on births in a year as appearing in the report on the 1974 Bangladesh Retrospective Survey of Fertility and Mortality.................... 41
11. Compilation of data on births in a year by age group of mother for Bangladesh 42

vii

INTRODUCTION

The aim of this *Guide* is to provide the reader with all the information necessary to apply two methods for the estimation of child mortality. It does not presuppose familiarity with demography or with basic demographic measures. The reader is introduced to the basic concepts encountered in the measurement of mortality, the typical indicators of mortality in childhood, the rationale underlying the methods described and the data required for their application. The procedures followed for the actual application of each method are described in step-by-step fashion, and some guidance is provided regarding the interpretation and use of the estimates obtained.

The *Guide* should be especially useful for persons who are engaged in programme activities aimed at reducing levels of infant and child mortality in developing countries and who require measures of such mortality to identify target population groups for whom mortality is high and to assess programme impact in terms of mortality reduction.

The conventional measurement of mortality requires information on the number of deaths and on the population subject to the risk of dying. Typically, the first type of information is derived from registration systems that record deaths as they occur; the second is obtained mostly from censuses. In the majority of developing countries, either registration systems do not exist or omission and other errors are so common that measures based on the data produced fail to reflect properly levels or trends of mortality.

Over the past twenty years, considerable advances have been made to compensate for the lack of reliable vital registration data. A number of methods based on information obtained exclusively from censuses or surveys have been developed, and census and survey data have become more commonly available. In this *Guide* two methods that use retrospective information on the children that women have borne will be described. The first, known as the Brass method (Brass, 1964), has proved to produce reliable estimates of child mortality in a variety of circumstances. The second, known as the Brass-Macrae method (Brass and Macrae, 1984), relies on information that can be obtained less expensively, and it promises to be useful in evaluating the impact of local projects. Because both of these methods rely on information that is only indirectly related to mortality, they are generally described as indirect estimation methods.

Other methods also exist for estimating child mortality, but they either require considerably more information than those described here or have proved less reliable. The reader interested in obtaining more information about such methods may consult the list of references in this *Guide*. Another useful source of information on indirect methods is chapter III of *Manual X: Indirect Techniques for Demographic Estimation* (United Nations, 1983b).

This *Guide* contains all the instructions necessary to apply two versions of the Brass method, named the Trussell and Palloni-Heligman versions after the persons who derived them, and another method, developed by Brass and Macrae. Since the *Guide* is intended for use by persons who need not have formal demographic training, it also includes an introduction to the basic demographic concepts involved in the estimation of mortality in childhood and detailed descriptions of the nature of the data required for each method.

The *Guide* is divided into seven chapters. The first discusses mortality measurement in general; the next five are devoted to different aspects of the Brass method; and the last focuses on the procedure proposed by Brass and Macrae. The Brass-Macrae method is treated in a single chapter because of both its relative simplicity and its recency. At the time of writing, the Brass-Macrae procedure is still in the process of being tested, and its efficacy cannot be guaranteed in all cases. The Brass method, on the other hand, has been used for more than two decades, has already given rise to numerous variations or refinements of the original procedure and, despite its known limitations, has performed well under a variety of circumstances. It is therefore recommended that every reader become acquainted with at least one version of the Brass method.

Although the material in this *Guide* has been presented in the simplest way possible, the *Guide's* content is not necessarily simple, and the reader should not expect to master it in a single reading. As with any learning process, an understanding of the intricacies of estimating mortality in childhood can be acquired only incrementally, by working and reworking through examples and by consulting several times the chapters discussing the rationale behind the different methods and their limitations.

To master the basics of the Brass method, it is recommended that the reader work through chapters I to IV in order. The aim should be to master chapters II and IV, on the data requirements of the Brass method and the application of one of its variants, while becoming familiar with mortality measurement in general as discussed in chapter I and with the strengths and limitations of the Brass method as presented in chapter III. Only after becoming thoroughly familiar with those chapters should the reader proceed to chapter V, in which a second version of the Brass method is described. Chapter VI, dealing with the interpretation and use of the estimates obtained, may be read early on, but the reader will find it more useful after chapters IV and V have been mastered.

Chapter VII, describing the Brass-Macrae method, may be studied almost independently from the rest, though it should not be read without some familiarity with the concepts presented in chapter I.

The *Guide* is accompanied by a program for microcomputers, named QFIVE, that applies both the Trussell and the Palloni-Heligman versions of the Brass method. Although the program can be used without a complete understanding of the Brass method, it is recommended that it be used only after mastering, at the very least, chapters II and IV. The computerized application of the estimation method is meant to free the analyst from the drudgery of longhand calculations, but it cannot replace the analyst's insight into the use and interpretation of the estimates obtained. Such insight can only be gained by understanding how a method works and why. The text of this *Guide* is meant to lead the reader to that understanding.

For the benefit of those interested in a more detailed description of the *Guide,* an annotated outline of its chapters follows.

Chapter I. *Indicators of mortality in childhood*

This chapter presents the demographic concepts used in the estimation of mortality in childhood. The life table, the basic demographic instrument for the measurement of mortality, is described in detail. Attention is then focused on the main indicators of mortality in childhood. The importance of considering mortality levels over the age range 0 to 5, rather than the age range 0 to 1, is explained. Through the discussion of model life table systems, the reader is introduced to different patterns of mortality in childhood. Examples of estimates for specific countries are used to illustrate the variety of existing patterns.

Chapter II. *Data required for the Brass method*

This chapter discusses in detail the data required to estimate mortality in childhood by using the Brass method. It provides worksheets to aid the user in compiling the data needed. By working through a detailed example, the user becomes familiar with possible variations of the basic data.

Chapter III. *Rationale of the Brass method*

This chapter describes heuristically the theoretical underpinnings of the Brass method and explains why the method works even under conditions of changing mortality. The limitations of the method and the possible biases that may result from violations of its basic assumptions are also discussed.

Chapter IV. *Trussell version of the Brass method*

This chapter describes, in step-by-step fashion, the application of one version of the Brass method, that proposed by Trussell. This version uses the Coale-Demeny model life tables, those most widely used to date. A detailed example and a brief discussion of the results provide the reader with practical information on the use of the method.

Chapter V. *Palloni-Heligman version of the Brass method*

This chapter describes a second version of the Brass method, that proposed by Palloni and Heligman. This version uses the United Nations model life tables for developing countries. Aside from describing the additional data that this procedure requires, the chapter provides a detailed example and briefly discusses the results obtained.

Chapter VI. *Interpretation and use of the estimates yielded by the Brass method*

This chapter compares the estimates obtained by using the Trussell and Palloni-Heligman versions of the Brass method. The problem of selecting an appropriate model life table is discussed, and the possible biases introduced by selecting the "wrong" model are assessed. In addition, the chapter considers the problem of comparing and assessing estimates obtained from different sources. Examples are given of how the estimates yielded by the Brass method can be used to determine mortality trends in childhood when data from difference sources are available.

Chapter VII. *Brass-Macrae method*

This chapter describes the basic data needed to apply the Brass-Macrae method, explains why it works and discusses its possible limitations. The procedure to apply the method is then described and illustrated with a detailed example. The results obtained are discussed in the light of the limited information available on the general performance of the method.

Chapter I

INDICATORS OF MORTALITY IN CHILDHOOD

LIFE TABLES

A life table is the demographer's way of representing the effects of mortality. A complete life table consists of several functions or sets of numbers, each representing a different aspect of the impact of mortality.[1] Table 1 provides an example of a life table. The core of the life table is the set of values shown in column 3 under the heading $1(x)$. Letting x denote age, those values represent the number of survivors by age out of an initial number of births (100,000 in table 1). Thus, according to the life table in table 1, out of 100,000 births, 86,874 persons survive to age 10 and 71,074 to age 50. These ages represent "exact ages", that is, the 71,074 survivors are persons alive at the exact moment at which they reach age 50: they are not a day older or a day younger than exact age 50.

The typical shape of the $1(x)$ function is displayed in the upper panel of figure 1. The number of survivors decreases markedly from birth (exact age 0) to ages 2 and 3 and then declines fairly slowly until around age 60, after which the decline accelerates.

The population for which the effects of mortality are represented by a life table is an example of a cohort. A cohort is a group of persons experiencing the same event during a given period. For instance, all persons marrying in 1974 constitute a marriage cohort. Similarly, all persons born in 1923 are a birth cohort. A life table represents the survivors of a birth cohort. However, the birth cohort represented by most life tables is not a real one, since it would not be possible to complete the life table until all the members of the birth cohort had died. For instance, a life table representing the survivors of the 1923 birth cohort could not be completed until some time around 2013 or 2023. Consequently, demographers resort to hypothetical birth cohorts, that is, cohorts that are a theoretical fabrication and that do not really exist. Thus, a period life table represents the effects of mortality on a hypothetical cohort that is assumed to be subject during its entire life to the mortality conditions prevalent during a given period.

Given the number of survivors of a hypothetical birth cohort by age—the $1(x)$ values—it is easy to calculate the number of deaths occurring from one age to the next.

TABLE 1.   EXAMPLE OF A LIFE TABLE

Age x (1)	n (2)	l(x) (3)	$_nd_x$ (4)	q_x (5)	$_nL_x$ (6)	$_nm_x$ (7)	e_x (8)
0	1	100 000	8 177	.0818	94 238	.0868	57.50
1	4	91 823	3 781	.0412	357 424	.0106	61.59
5	5	88 041	1 167	.0133	437 289	.0027	60.18
10	5	86 874	894	.0103	432 136	.0021	55.96
15	5	85 980	1 277	.0149	426 708	.0030	51.51
20	5	84 703	1 651	.0195	419 388	.0039	47.25
25	5	83 052	1 858	.0224	410 617	.0045	43.14
30	5	81 194	2 075	.0256	400 784	.0052	39.07
35	5	79 119	2 321	.0293	389 794	.0060	35.03
40	5	76 798	2 624	.0342	377 432	.0070	31.01
45 ...,...........	5	74 175	3 100	.0418	363 122	.0085	27.02
50	5	71 074	4 059	.0571	345 223	.0118	23.09
55	5	67 015	5 250	.0783	321 951	.0163	19.34
60	5	61 765	7 226	.1170	290 761	.0249	15.77
65	5	54 539	9 389	.1722	249 225	.0377	12.53
70	5	45 151	11 799	.2613	196 255	.0601	9.61
75	5	33 352	12 807	.3840	13 474	.0951	7.13
80	20	20 545	20 545	1.0000	102 911	.1996	5.01

Source: Ansley J. Coale and Paul Demeny, *Regional Model Life Tables and Stable Populations* (Princeton, Princeton University Press, 1966, p.17

$l(x)$ number of survivors to exact age x

$_nd_x$ number of deaths between exact ages x and $x + n$

$_nq_x$ probability of dying between exact ages x and $x + n$

$_nL_x$ number of person-years lived between exact ages x and $x + n$

$_nm_x$ age-specific mortality rate for age group x to $x + n$

e_x expectation of life at exact age x

Figure 1.   Typical shapes of the $l(x)$ and $_1q_x$ functions of a life table

Survivors of 100,000 female births by age, 1(x)
Thousands of survivors
100
90
80
70
60
50
40
30
20
10
0
10
20
30
40
50
60
70
80
90
Age

Probability of dying at each age, $_1q_x$
Probability of dying
.20
.18
.16
.14
.12
.10
.08
.06
.04
.02
0
10
20
30
40
50
60
70
80
90
Age

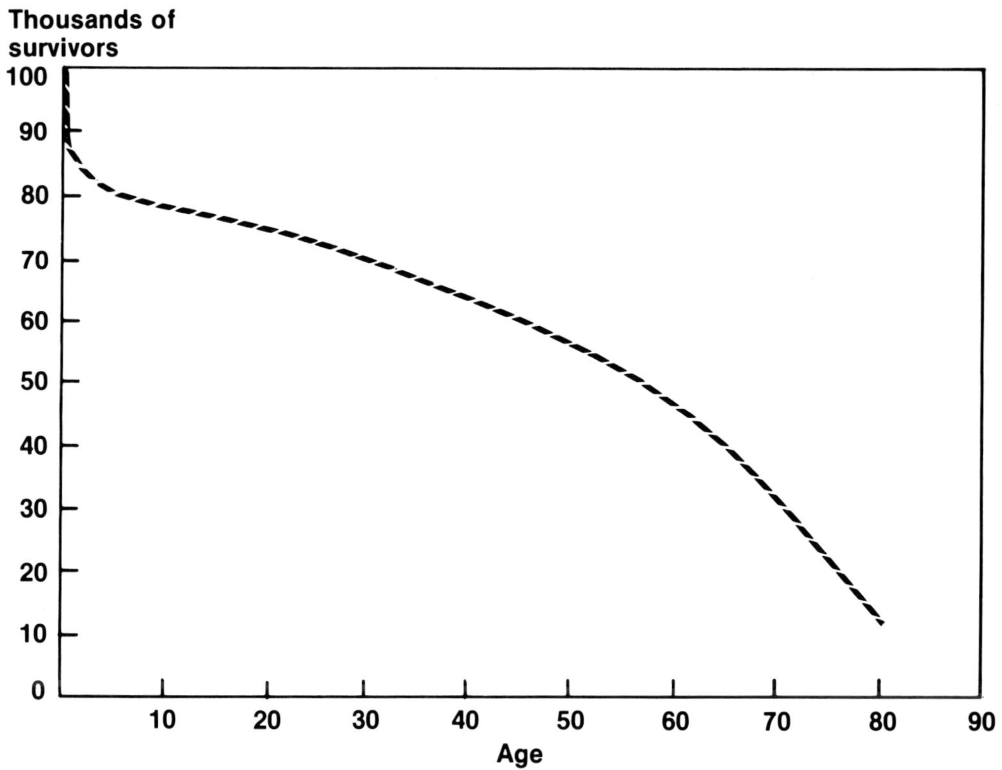

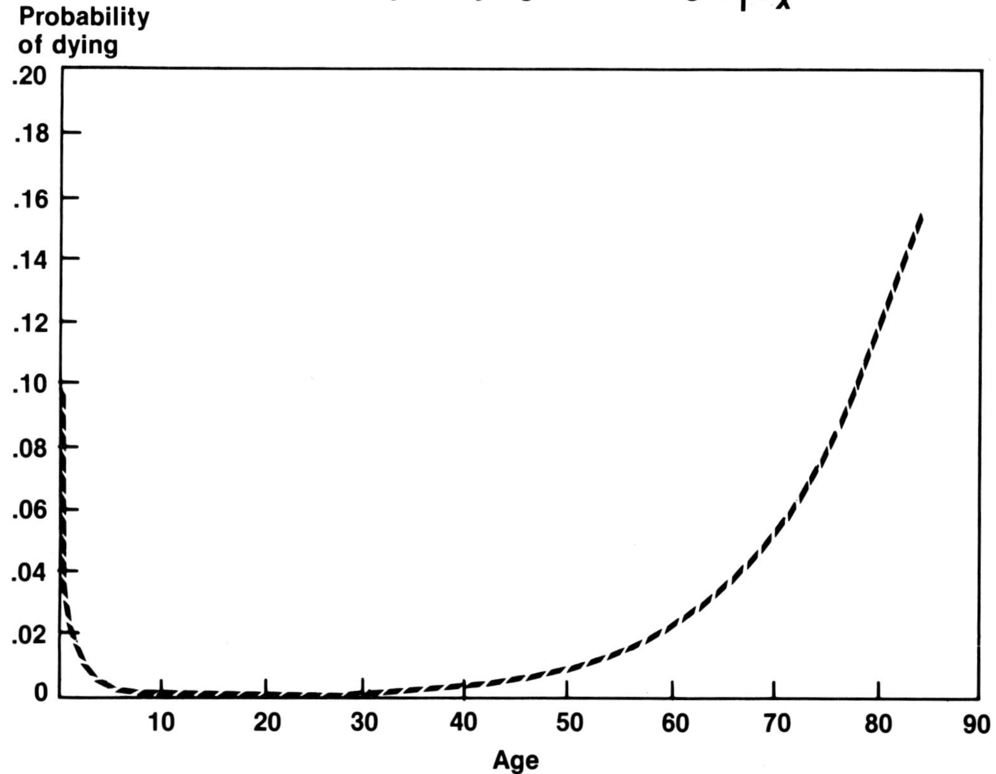

4

Consider ages 20 and 25. In the life table displayed in table 1, 1(20)—the number of survivors to age 20—is 84,703, and 1(25)—the number of survivors to age 25—is 83,052. Hence, the number of persons dying between ages 20 and 25 equals the difference between those numbers, that is, $84,703 - 83,052 = 1,651$. Note that the number 1,651 appears in the line corresponding to age 20 under the column headed $_nd_x$, a notation that stands for the number of deaths occurring between ages x and $x + n$. Thus, $_5d_{20} = 1,651$. All the other numbers in column 4 of table 1 are calculated in the same way.

Once the number of deaths occurring in the hypothetical birth cohort in each age interval is known, the probability of dying in each age interval can be calculated. For instance, if 1,651 deaths occur among the 84,703 survivors to age 20 during the next five years of their lives, the probability of each dying before reaching age 25 is $1,651/84,703 = .0195$. The number .0195 appears in the line for age 20 of the life table under the column headed $_nq_x$, which is the actuarial notation for the probability of dying between ages x and $x + n$.

The lower panel of figure 1 illustrates the typical shape of the probability of dying at each age, $_1q_x$. Note that the probability of dying is generally high among children under age 5, and especially among children under age 1 (i.e. infants). It falls to a minimum around age 10 and rises gradually up to age 50 or so. Thereafter it rises steeply until very high levels are reached in old age.

Although this *Guide* is concerned mainly with the estimation of probabilities of dying between birth and certain ages in childhood, $_nq_0$, it is worth defining here the rest of the life-table functions, which are displayed in table 1. Their derivation requires the introduction of a new concept: the time lived by survivors between exact ages.

Consider again the interval between exact ages 20 and 25 and note that $l(20)$ is 84,703 and $l(25)$ is 83,052 (that is, out of 100,000 persons born alive, 84,703 survive to exact age 20 and 83,052 survive to exact age 25). Clearly, each of the 83,052 survivors to age 25 lives five years between exact ages 20 and 25, for a total of 5 × 83,052 = 415,260 years lived. However, the 1,651 persons who die also contribute some years lived to the total. Assuming, for simplicity's sake, that all those who die do so at the midpoint of the interval—that is, at exact age 22.5—each one therefore contributes 2.5 years of life, for an additional 2.5 × 1,651 = 4,128 years lived. Hence, the total number of years lived between exact ages 20 and 25 by the hypothetical cohort under consideration is the sum of those quantities—419,388. This value is denoted by $_5L_{20}$ and, in general, the $_nL_x$ function represents the number of person-years lived by the hypothetical life-table cohort between exact ages x and $x + n$.

The $_nL_x$ function is the basis for the calculation of a valuable summary measure of mortality conditions, the expectation of life at birth. If the $_nL_x$ values are cumulated from birth to the highest age to which anyone survives—say 100—the resulting sum will be the total number of years lived by the hypothetical life-table cohort during its lifetime. The average number of years

lived by each member of that cohort will then be that total divided by the initial cohort size (the radix, denoted by $l(0)$). Such an average is known as the expectation of life at birth, e_0, an index that summarizes mortality conditions at all ages. In table 1 the last column shows values of the e_x function, that is, the expectation of life at exact age x. The first value is e_0; the others represent the average number of additional years of life expected by each of the survivors to exact age x.

The $_nL_x$ function also allows the calculation of another important set of mortality measures: age-specific death or mortality rates. Death rates measure the velocity at which deaths occur in a given population through time. Their numerator is the number of deaths observed at a given age or for a given age group during a certain period, and their denominator is the time or duration of exposure to the risk of dying experienced during that period by the population being considered. In the case of a life-table cohort, the time of exposure to the risk of dying is provided by the number of person-years lived between one exact age and another, that is, by the $_nL_x$ function. Hence, the death rate between ages x and $x + n$, denoted by $_nm_x$, is defined as

$$_nm_x = \frac{_nd_x}{_nL_x} \qquad (1.1)$$

Put another way, $_nm_x$ is the number of deaths of persons aged x to $x + n$ per person-year lived by the hypothetical life-table cohort between those ages. Note that this measure is intrinsically different from $_nq_x$, which represents the number of deaths of persons aged x to $x + n$ per surviving person at age x. In other words, death rates are measures of deaths per unit of time of exposure, whereas probabilities of dying are measures of deaths per person exposed. As columns 5 and 7 of table 1 show, the quantitative difference between the two measures is substantial, largely because $_nm_x$ is a rate per person-year while $_nq_x$ is generally a probability over a period of five years.

MEASUREMENT OF MORTALITY IN CHILDHOOD

The estimation of mortality in childhood has traditionally focused on mortality below age 1 because, as shown in figure 1, mortality at early ages is highest among infants (persons under age 1) and because measures of mortality for the age range 0 to 1 can be obtained solely from registration data when those data are reliable.

However, given the lack of reliable registration data in most developing countries and the widespread use of indirect methods to estimate mortality in childhood, attention has slowly shifted to the measurement of mortality over an expanded range in childhood. Thus, UNICEF has recently been publishing sets of estimates of mortality in childhood that include not only infant mortality, $_1q_0$, but also under-five mortality, $_5q_0$, for all the countries of the world (see, for instance, UNICEF, 1986, 1987a, 1987b, 1988a, and 1988b). Such a shift has come about mainly for two reasons: first, the realization that in many countries mortality levels among children older than 1 can be substantial, and, second, the fact that the most widely used indirect method of estimating mortality in child-

5

hood, the Brass method, produces more reliable estimates of under-five mortality than of infant mortality.

Note that the indices used by UNICEF are probabilities of dying between certain ages: infant mortality is the probability of dying between birth and exact age 1, $_1q_0$; child mortality is the probability of dying between exact ages 1 and 5, $_4q_1$; and under-five mortality is the probability of dying between birth and exact age 5, $_5q_0$. Throughout this *Guide* probabilities are used as indicators of mortality in childhood. To simplify notation, probabilities of dying between birth and exact age x, instead of being denoted by the standard notation, $_xq_0$, are denoted by $q(x)$. Note, however, that in referring to the probability of dying between exact ages 1 and 5, also known as child mortality, the traditional notation $_4q_1$ will be used, since the age span in this case does not start at birth.

To give the reader an idea of the values that infant and under-five mortality estimates may take, table 2 shows average estimates and projections of mortality in childhood for the major regions of the world during the periods 1950-1955, 1965-1970 and 1980-1985. Note that the more developed regions exhibit consistently lower infant and under-five mortality than do developing regions. Africa, in particular, is characterized by very high mortality in childhood. Recent estimates prepared by the United Nations Population Division (United Nations, 1988) show that infant mortality, $q(1)$, currently varies from a low of 6 deaths per 1,000 live births to a high of over 150 deaths per 1,000. Under-five mortality, $q(5)$, varies between 7 and over 250 deaths per 1,000 live births. Hence, in countries with the highest mortality, slightly more than one out of every six children dies before the age of 1 and one out of every four dies before reaching age 5.

COHORT VERSUS PERIOD MEASURES OF MORTALITY IN CHILDHOOD

It was stated earlier that, in constructing life tables, demographers often use hypothetical cohorts because of the practical constraints inherent in following a real birth cohort through its entire life. However, when the age span of interest corresponds to childhood only or, more specifically, is the age range 0 to 5, the drawbacks of dealing with real cohorts are less serious. Consequently, measures of mortality in childhood referring to real cohorts, called cohort measures, are relatively common in the literature. In order to interpret such measures correctly, the reader should be aware of how cohort measures differ from period measures, which refer to hypothetical cohorts that reflect the mortality conditions prevalent during a given period (a year in most instances).

Consider the problem of counting the deaths occurring before age 1 to the cohort born in 1979. Since the dates of birth of the members of that cohort are likely to span the whole range of dates between 1 January 1979 and 31 December 1979, in order to count all deaths before age 1, it is necessary to observe the cohort from 1 January 1979, when its first members are born, to 31 December 1980, when its last members become 1. In other words, a two-year observation period is necessary to estimate the incidence of mortality among cohort members aging, on average, one year.

Now suppose that, rather than being interested in the deaths occurring in a particular birth cohort, one wants to know how mortality affects persons under age 1 in a particular year, say 1980. Note that persons under 1 in 1980 include not only those born between 1 January and 31 December 1980, who will clearly be under age 1 during the whole year, but also those born in 1979 who will be under age 1 during at least part of 1980. Thus, to measure mortality among persons under age 1 in 1980, information is needed on deaths occurring in 1980 among members of two birth cohorts: that born in 1979 and that born in 1980.

The Lexis diagram (figure 2) provides a graphic illustration of the relation between cohort and period measures. The horizontal axis of the diagram represents time in calendar years, while the vertical axis represents age. Then, the diagonal lines in the diagram represent the trajectory of persons as they age. Thus, the line AE

TABLE 2. ESTIMATES OF THE PROBABILITIES OF DYING BY AGES 1 AND 5, $q(1)$ AND $q(5)$, BY MAJOR REGION, 1950-1955, 1965-1970 AND 1980-1985

Major region	Probability of dying by age 1 (per 1,000 births)			Probability of dying by age 5 (per 1,000 births)		
	1950-1955	1965-1970	1980-1985	1950-1955	1965-1970	1980-1985
World	156	103	78	240	161	118
More developed regions	56	26	16	73	32	19
Less developed regions	180	117	88	281	184	134
Africa	191	158	112	322	261	182
Latin America	125	91	62	189	131	88
Northern America	29	22	11	34	26	13
East Asia	182	76	36	248	106	50
South Asia	180	135	103	305	219	157
Europe	62	30	15	77	35	17
Oceania	67	48	31	96	67	40
Union of Soviet Socialist Republics	73	26	25	102	36	31

Source: *Mortality of Children under age 5: World Estimates and Projections, 1950-2025,* Population Studies, No.105 (United Nations publication, Sales No. E.88.XIII.4).

represents persons born on 1 January 1979 who reach age 1 on 1 January 1980, while line BF represents persons born on 31 December 1979 who reach age 1 on 31 December 1980. That is, the parallelogram AEFB represents the cohort born in 1979 as it ages from 0 to 1. Since squares of the type BEFC represent yearly periods, it can be seen that, as the 1979 cohort ages, it spans parts of the 1979 and 1980 periods. Conversely, in the 1980 period (BEFC), parts of two cohorts find themselves in the age range 0 to 1: the one born in 1979 and represented by the triangle BEF and that born in 1980, whose triangle is BFC. Thus, the deaths of children under age 1 in 1980 comprise deaths of some children born in 1979 and of some born in 1980.

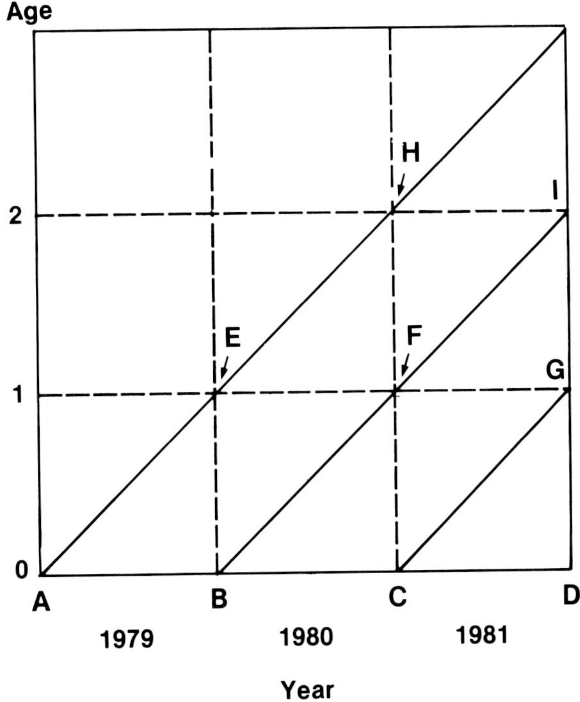

Figure 2. Relation between cohort and period measures shown by a Lexis diagram

This example illustrates how period measures represent the combined experience of different birth cohorts, whereas cohort measures represent the combined experience of cohort measures during different periods. The Lexis diagram illustrates this by showing how the cohort diagonals cut across periods while the vertical bars representing periods cut across different cohorts.

In this *Guide,* the aim is to obtain period measures of mortality in all instances. However, to understand how those measures are derived, it is often necessary to consider the interplay between cohort and period indices.

MODEL LIFE TABLES

In many countries where death registration is incomplete or non-existent, adequate life tables cannot be constructed from the available data. Indeed, little may be known about the actual age pattern of mortality of their populations. Model life tables, which represent expected age patterns of mortality, have been developed for use in such cases.

A number of model-life-table systems exist, but in this *Guide* only two will be used, the Coale-Demeny regional model life tables (Coale and Demeny, 1983) and the United Nations model life tables for developing countries (United Nations, 1982).

The Coale-Demeny life tables consist of four sets or models, each representing a distinct mortality pattern. Each model is arranged in terms of 25 mortality levels, associated with different expectations of life at birth for females in such a way that e_0 of 20 years corresponds to level 1 and e_0 of 80 years corresponds to level 25. The four underlying mortality patterns of the Coale-Demeny models are called "North", "South", "East" and "West". They were identified through statistical and graphical analysis of a large number of life tables of acceptable quality, mainly for European countries.

The United Nations models encompass five distinct mortality patterns, known as "Latin American", "Chilean", "South Asian", "Far Eastern" and "General". Life tables representative of each pattern are arranged by expectations of life at birth ranging from 35 to 75 years. The different patterns were identified through statistical and graphical analysis of a number of evaluated and adjusted life tables for developing countries.

Model life tables play a crucial role in the estimation of mortality in childhood. They underlie the derivation of the estimation methods themselves and serve in evaluating the results obtained. Thus, to make proper use of model life tables in estimating child mortality, it is necessary to be familiar with the characteristic patterns that they embody, especially at younger ages. Figures 3 and 4 show one way of comparing those patterns. In both graphs the values of infant mortality, $q(1)$ (the probability of dying by exact age 1), have been plotted against the values of child mortality, $_4q_1$ (the probability of dying between exact ages 1 and 5), for each model. Thus, each curve in figures 3 and 4 represents the typical relationship between infant and child mortality in a given life table model.

With respect to the Coale-Demeny models for both males and females, figure 3 shows that for any given value of $q(1)$ above .15, model East produces the lowest mortality between ages 1 and 5, $_4q_1$, followed by West and then North. Model South's pattern at young ages overlaps that of East for very low values of $q(1)$, crosses that of West for intermediate values and goes beyond that of North at high values of infant mortality. In other words, model East is appropriate for populations where the risks of dying between ages 1 and 5 are low with respect to those of dying in infancy, whereas model North is appropriate when the former are high with respect to the latter. Model West, falling in between those two, is a good compromise as an "average" model.

Figure 4 shows the equivalent comparisons for the United Nations models. Notice that, in contrast with the Coale-Demeny models, the curves do not intersect and that the order of the models varies by sex. However, the proximity of the curves corresponding to all the patterns

Figure 3.   Relationship between infant mortality, $q(1)$, and
child mortality, $_4q_1$, in the Coale-Demeny mortality models

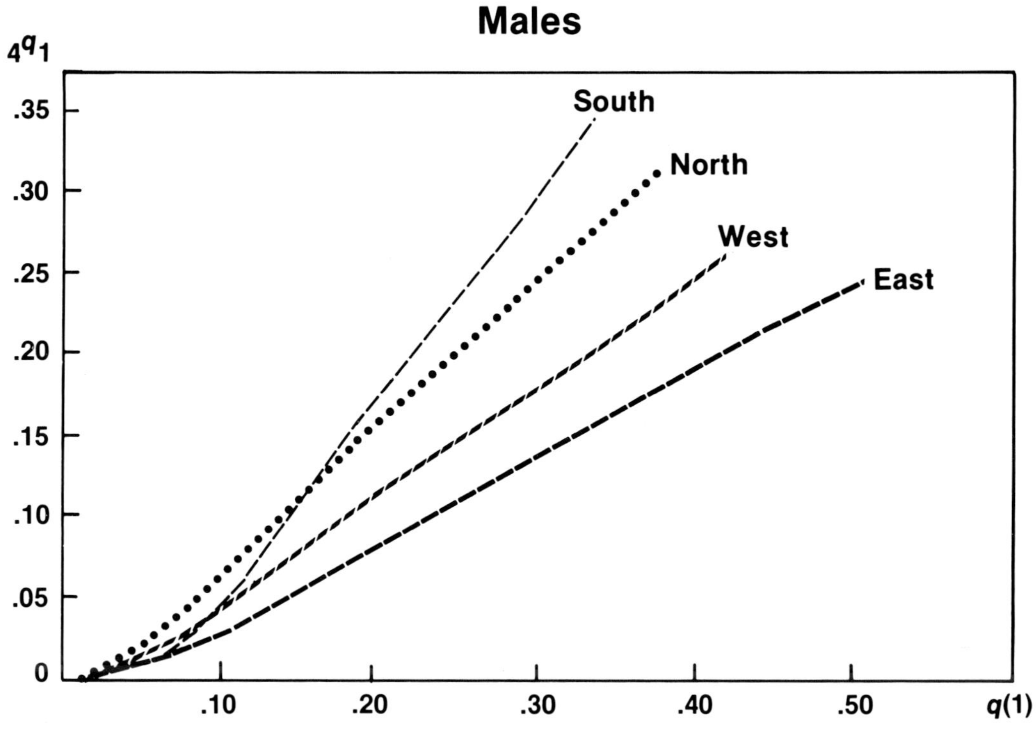

Males
$_4q_1$
.35
.30
.25
.20
.15
.10
.05
0
South
North
West
East
.10
.20
.30
.40
.50
q(1)

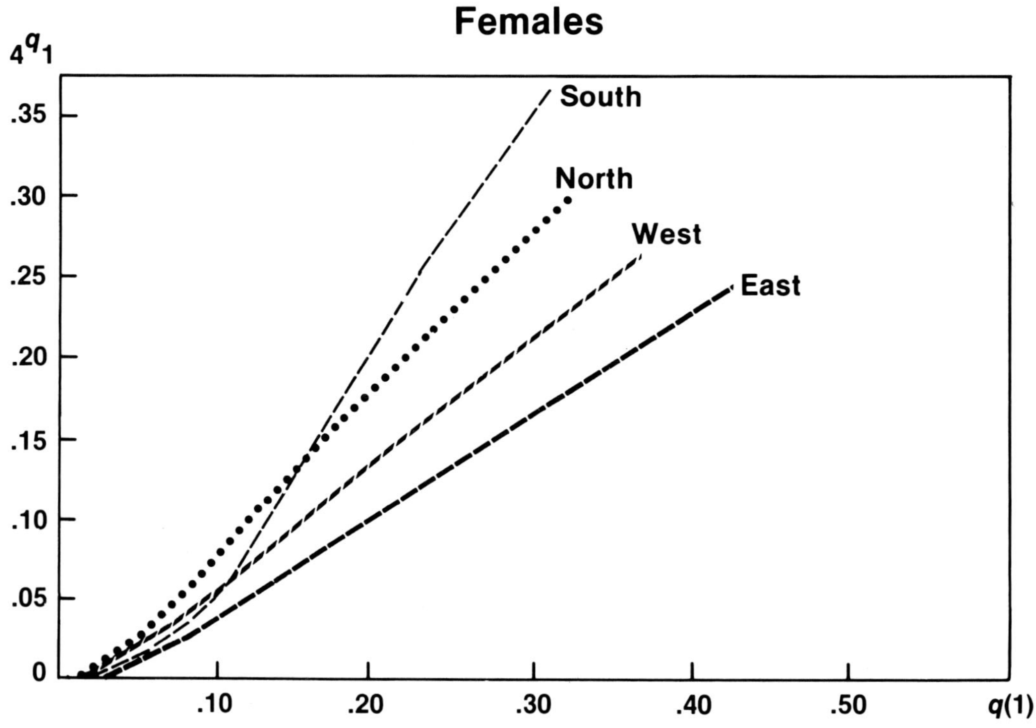

Females
$_4q_1$
.35
.30
.25
.20
.15
.10
.05
0
South
North
West
East
.10
.20
.30
.40
.50
q(1)

Figure 4. Relationship between infant mortality, $q(1)$, and child mortality, $_4q_1$, in the United Nations mortality models

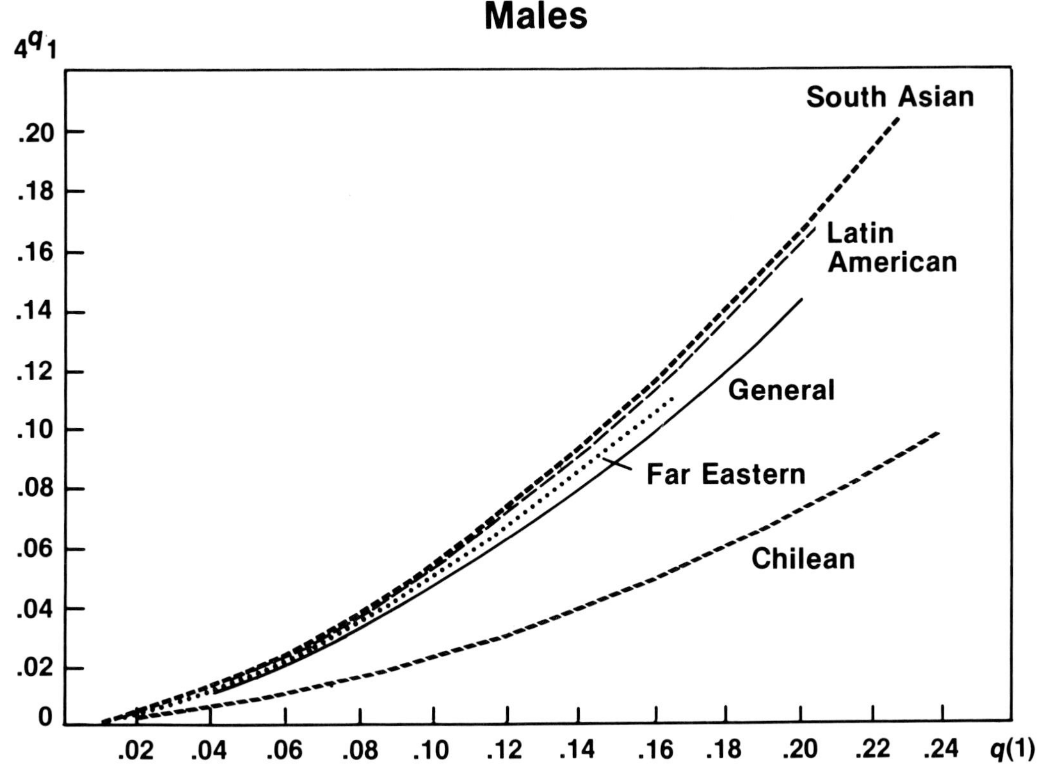

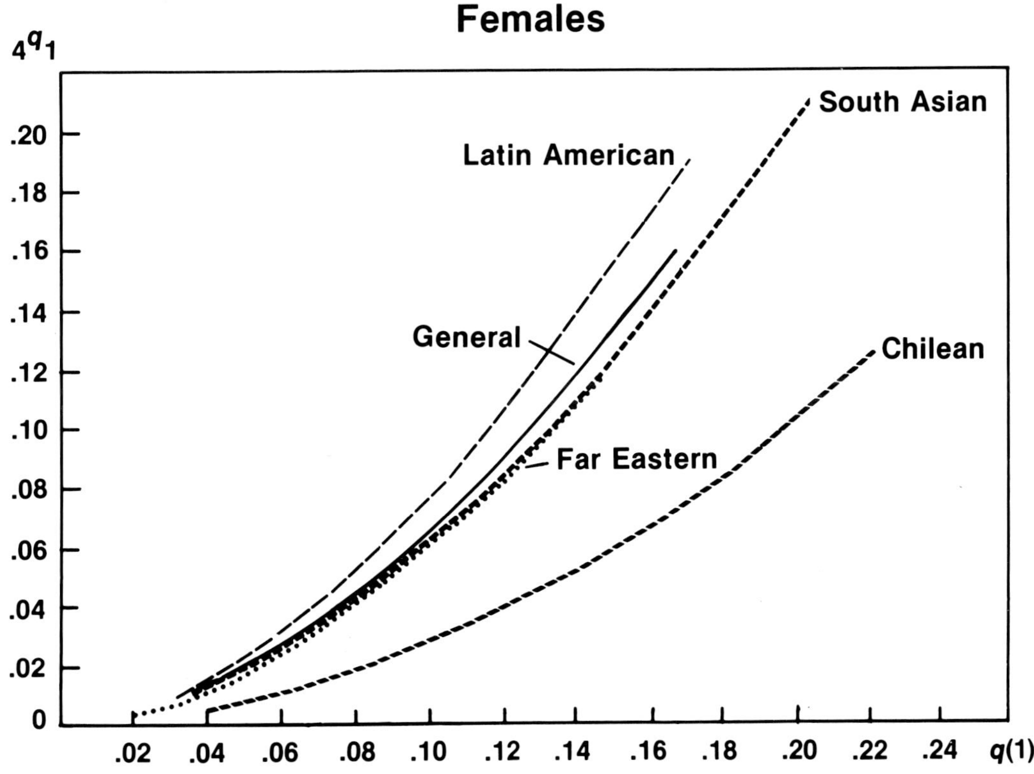

except the Chilean one implies that the United Nations models are less differentiated at younger ages than the Coale-Demeny models. The marked differences existing between the Chilean pattern and all the others should be noted, especially since the Chilean pattern is "more East than East", in that it represents the experience of a population whose mortality risks between ages 1 and 5 are very low compared with those below age 1.

The importance of these models and their distinctive traits will become evident during the description and use of the methods presented below. Those interested in obtaining a more detailed description of model life tables in general may consult chapter I of *Manual X: Indirect Techniques for Demographic Estimation* (United Nations, 1983b), chapters 1 and 2 of *Regional Model Life Tables and Stable Populations* (Coale and Demeny, 1983) and chapters I to IV of *Model Life Tables for Developing Countries* (United Nations, 1982).

OBSERVED PATTERNS OF MORTALITY IN CHILDHOOD
AND THE MODEL LIFE TABLES

To give the reader a sense of how well the mortality models available reflect the actual experience of different populations, figures 5 and 6 compare the relationship

Figure 5. Comparison of country-specific estimates of infant and child mortality
with the Coale-Demeny mortality models

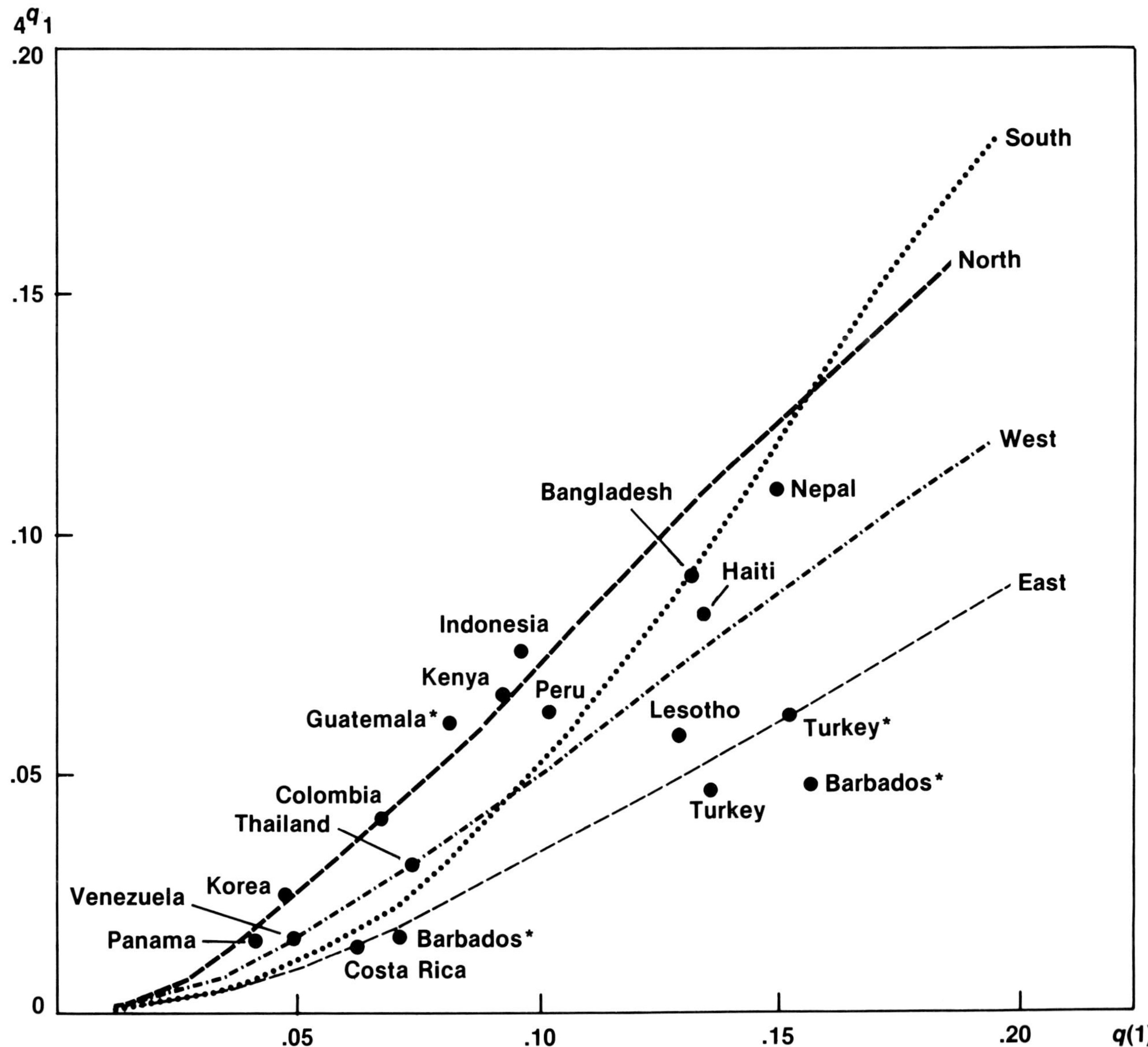

Sources: For most countries, the estimates shown are those referring to the period 0-9 years before the World Fertility Survey and published in Shea O. Rutstein, *Infant and Child Mortality: Levels, Trends and Demographic Differentials,* Comparative Studies, No. 24 (London, World Fertility Survey, 1983); the upper right estimate for Turkey was obtained from a multiround survey (1966-1967 Turkish Demographic Survey); the estimates for Barbados were calculated from vital registration data referring to 1945-1947 (upper right) and 1959-1961 (lower left); for Guatemala the estimates used refer to 1975-1980 (see *Mortality of Children under Age 5: World Estimates and Projections, 1950-2025,* Population Studies, No. 105 (United Nations publication, Sales No. E.88.XIII.4). For the mortality models (North, South, East, West), see Ansley J. Coale and Paul Demeny, *Regional Model Life Tables and Stable Populations* (Princeton, Princeton University Press, 1966).

*Estimates obtained from sources other than the World Fertility Survey.

between the infant and child mortality typical of the different model life tables with that observed in selected countries. The data for most of the countries depicted were derived from the set of World Fertility Surveys carried out during the second half of the 1970s. The estimates for Barbados and Guatemala and one of the estimates for Turkey were obtained from other sources.

For the most part, the estimates of $q(1)$ and $_4q_1$ plotted in figures 5 and 6 were derived from the fertility histories of women interviewed. A fertility history is the series of dates of birth and, if appropriate, dates of death of all the children a woman has had. The estimates of $q(1)$ and $_4q_1$ used here were obtained from the births and deaths of children under age 5 occurring during the 10 years preceding each survey.

Bearing in mind that the accuracy and reliability of the country estimates displayed in figures 5 and 6 may vary, it is useful to consider the degree to which they can be approximated by existing mortality models. Figure 5 shows that the Coale-Demeny models provide excellent approximations for a few countries: Colombia is North, Thailand and Venezuela are West, Bangladesh is South, and Costa Rica and the upper point for Turkey are East. For a few other countries, the models provide very good

Figure 6. Comparison of country-specific estimates of infant and child mortality with the United Nations mortality models

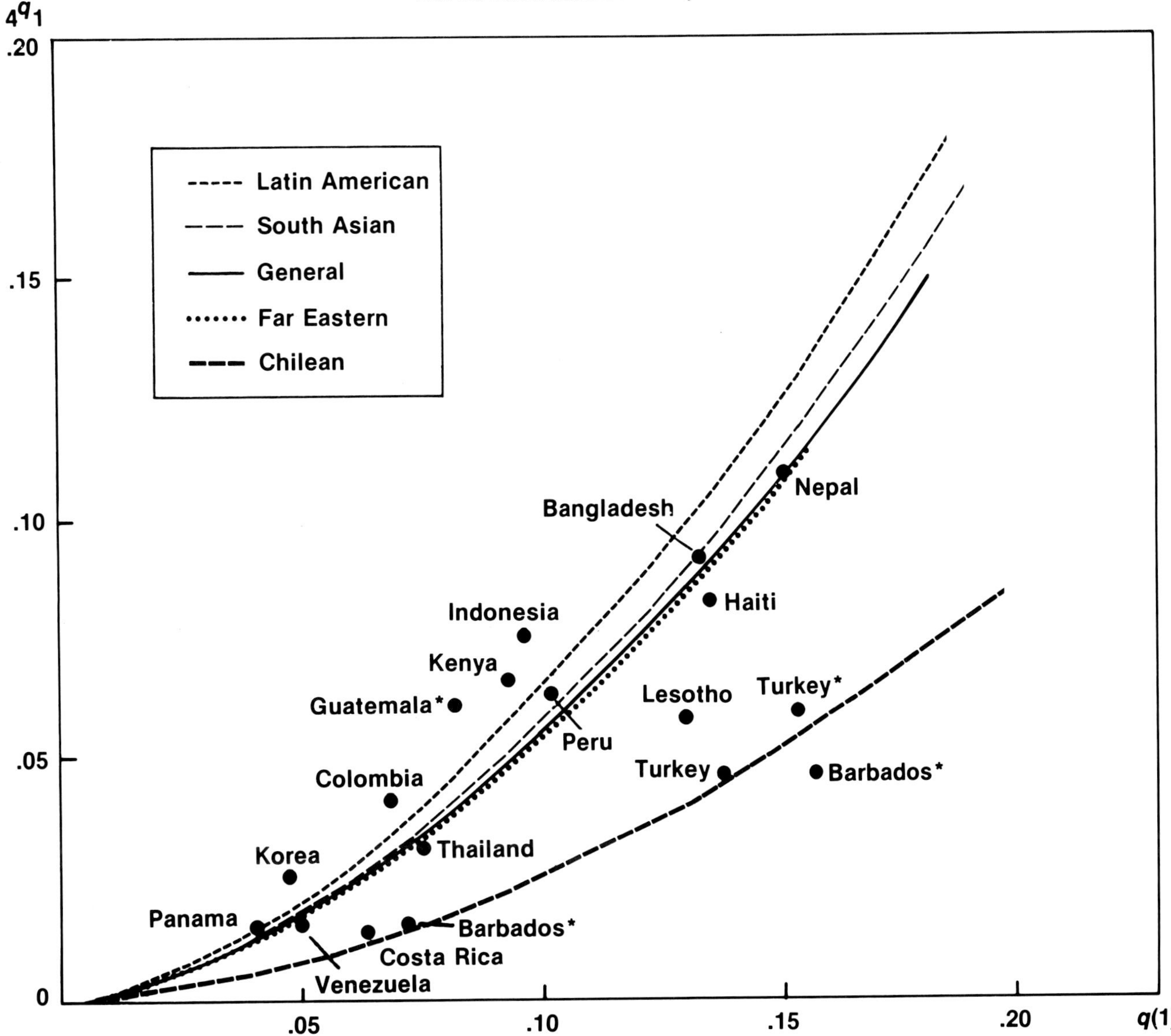

Sources: For most countries, the estimates shown are those referring to the period 0-9 years before the World Fertility Survey and published in Shea O. Rutstein, *Infant and Child Mortality: Levels, Trends and Demographic Differentials,* Comparative Studies, No. 24 (London, World Fertility Survey, 1983); the upper right estimate for Turkey was obtained from a multiround survey (1966-1967 Turkish Demographic Survey); the estimates for Barbados were calculated from vital registration data referring to 1945-1947 (upper right) and 1959-1961 (lower left); for Guatemala the estimates used refer to 1975-1980 (see *Mortality of Children under Age 5: World Estimates and Projections, 1950-2025,* Population Studies, No. 105 (United Nations publication, Sales No. E.88.XIII.4). For the mortality models (Latin American, Chilean, South Asian, Far Eastern and General), see *Model Life Tables for Developing Countries,* Population Studies, No. 77 (United Nations publication, Sales No. E.81.XIII.7).

*Estimates obtained from sources other than the World Fertility Survey.

11

approximations: Korea, Panama and Kenya are close to North, and the lower point for Barbados is close to East. There are other countries, however, for which the approximation provided by the Coale-Demeny models is less satisfactory, though compromises may be reached if a single model needs to be selected to represent each of them. Thus, for instance, Guatemala and Indonesia may be approximated by model North; Peru and Nepal by South; Haiti by West; and Lesotho, the lower point for Turkey and the upper point for Barbados by East.

Figure 6 shows the same comparison between the United Nations models and country-specific estimates. It is interesting to note that some of the countries that were fit very well by the Coale-Demeny models are no longer close to any United Nations model (for instance, Korea, Colombia and Kenya). On the other hand, some countries whose estimates are relatively far from the Coale-Demeny models are close to certain United Nations models (e.g., Nepal fits the General pattern and Turkey is close to the Chilean). Among the rest of the countries considered, the majority can be fit relatively well by either the Coale-Demeny or the United Nations models, though in particular instances one set of models provides a better fit than the other. Thus, while Costa Rica appears to be exactly East and Venezuela and Thailand are clearly West, Panama is Latin American. There remain, however, countries that are not adequately approximated by any of the models used here. Indonesia, Guatemala, Lesotho and the upper point for Barbados are some examples. To a lesser extent, Peru and Haiti also belong to that group, although they are closer to the United Nations models than to the Coale-Demeny models.

These comparisons show that the models generally provide good fits for the data observed on actual populations. However, and perhaps not surprisingly, the real world exhibits greater variety than is captured by available models. Even though some of the differences between the models and country-specific estimates may arise from errors in the basic data, it is certain that different mortality patterns exist. As will be seen, one of the challenges in using the Brass method is to make allowance for the appropriate mortality pattern in each case.

Chapter II

DATA REQUIRED FOR THE BRASS METHOD

At least since the 1940s, demographers working in developing countries have been aware that the proportion of children dead among those ever borne by women in a given age group is an indicator of mortality in childhood. The actual proportion observed is known to be largely determined by two factors: the mortality risks to which children are exposed and the duration of exposure to those risks. In 1964 William Brass proposed a method that permitted the estimation of mortality risks by making allowance for the duration of exposure, and thus it became possible to derive estimates of various values of $q(x)$—the probability of dying between birth and exact age x—from the observed proportions of children dead.

As suggested above, data on children ever born and children dead were available in some developing countries long before an estimation method was devised. Even today, the power of the Brass method stems not only from its theoretical underpinnings but also from its use of data that are relatively easy to obtain and whose reliability is generally acceptable. As with any other estimation method, the quality of the basic data used as input largely determines the quality of the resulting estimates. It is essential, therefore, to ensure that the highest standards are adhered to at all stages of data-gathering.

Although this *Guide* does not purport to be a manual for data collection, it is important for the analyst to have a clear grasp of what is being measured and of how different questions can be used to best advantage. Not only is such understanding necessary to avoid errors in the application of the estimation method, it is also an asset in evaluating the estimates obtained.

Nature of the data required

In its simplest variant, the Brass method requires three pieces of information: the number of children ever born, the number of children ever born who have died (children dead) and the total female population of reproductive age.

Children ever born and children dead

The information on children ever born and dead is normally obtained as follows. In a survey or census, women in a given age range (15 to 49, usually) are asked a certain number of questions about their child-bearing experience. The sets of questions that may be used include:

Set 1. How many children, who were born alive, have you ever had?
How many of those children have died?

Set 2. How many children, who were born alive, have you ever had?
How many are still alive?

Set 3. How many living children do you have?
How many children have you had who were born alive and later died?

Set 4. How many children do you have who live with you?
How many children do you have who live elsewhere?
How many children have you had who were born alive and later died?

Notice that the answers to each set of questions will yield, in some cases by addition or subtraction, the number of children ever born and the number of children dead that each woman has had. Notice also that only those children who were born alive should be counted as "children ever born". Abortions and, particularly, still-births should not be included.

Among the sets of questions presented, set 4 is generally considered to produce the best results, because, by focusing attention on both the children present and those absent, it leads to a lower level of omission. Set 3 is also recommended because, by avoiding the direct use of the concept of "children ever born", it may be easier for the respondent to grasp. Sets 1 and 2 may yield imperfect data when respondents fail to understand that children dead should also be reported as ever born. They may also lead to errors in societies where the qualifier "born alive" is construed to mean "still living". However, in societies where explicit mention of dead children is not acceptable, set 2 may provide the best means of gathering the required information.

In some surveys or censuses, the sets of questions presented here are posed separately with respect to male and female children. Data on children ever born and dead by sex are useful not only because they allow the estimation of mortality by sex, but also because they permit further evaluation of the quality of the data, as will be explained later on.

Certain surveys may produce data on children ever born and dead by gathering information on the fertility history of each woman. Roughly speaking, such information consists of the dates of birth of all children a woman has had and the dates of death of all deceased children. Complete fertility histories allow the calculation of the total number of children ever born and dead for each woman and thus permit the application of the Brass method. They also allow the application of other procedures to estimate child mortality and consequently provide several opportunities to check the internal consistency of the data. However, fertility histories involve considerable data-collection efforts and are very costly. For that reason, they are not considered typical data sources for the information needed to apply the Brass method.

Being aware of the variety of ways in which information on children ever born and dead may be gathered is important because the analyst must be prepared to convert existing tabulations of the actual items of information collected by censuses or surveys into the format required for estimation. Although those data are often tabulated according to such characteristics as labour-force participation or education of women—which may allow the analysis of differentials of mortality in childhood by socio-economic indicators—the Brass method requires only that data on children ever born and dead be classified by age of mother. The traditional five-year age groups—15-19, 20-24, 25-29, 30-34, 35-39, 40-44 and 45-49—are typically used for tabulation purposes and produce the data needed for the estimation method.

Total female population of reproductive age

Turning now to the third item of information needed for the estimation procedure—the total female population of reproductive age (15-49)—the reader must be warned that it is a source of multiple errors. Problems arise because the method assumes that the data used are representative of all women aged 15 to 49, irrespective of their child-bearing or marital status. In practice, some women fail to provide the information sought, thus becoming cases of "non-response". More importantly, some women are purposefully excluded from providing information, as in countries where it is considered inappropriate to ask single women about their child-bearing experience. Yet, tabulations of the data on children ever born and dead usually include a column headed "total number of women", often without explicitly indicating that only women actually providing information are included. Mistakes arise when those numbers of women are used in the application of the method, which requires that all women, irrespective of whether they provided information, be considered.

COMPILATION OF THE DATA REQUIRED

Although, as stated earlier, the Brass method requires a minimum of information—the number of children ever born, the number of children dead and the total female population of reproductive age—that information is collected and published in a variety of ways.[2] To aid the analyst in compiling and organizing the data required, two worksheets have been prepared (displays 1 and 2). The worksheets show items of information often found in actual tabulations. The analyst can obtain the information necessary to apply the Brass method by addition and subtraction (the appropriate combination or combinations of items are indicated in the heading of each column).

Note that the worksheets make allowance for the availability of information by sex, although data for both sexes combined are all that is needed. As indicated above, when data by sex are available, not only can mortality be estimated for each sex separately, but also the internal consistency of the information can be checked by calculating the ratios of male to female children ever born. Those ratios are estimates of the sex ratio at birth, that is, the average number of male births per female birth. That number is a biological constant that varies little from population to population and is generally found within the range of 1.03 to 1.08 male births per female birth. As the example in chapter IV will show, values of the sex ratio at birth that deviate markedly from the range of expected values indicate possible deficiencies in the basic data.

THE CASE OF BANGLADESH

The case of Bangladesh will be used as an example in the application of two versions of the Brass method, so it is appropriate to consider here the nature of the data available for that country. In 1974 a Retrospective Survey of Fertility and Mortality conducted in Bangladesh included questions on children ever born and children dead. Display 3 reproduces the tabulation of such information appearing in the published report. From that tabulation it can be inferred that questions such as those constituting set 4 (see p. 13) were used to gather the basic information and that they were posed only to ever-married women (that is, single women were not even asked the questions). Consequently, although the second column is labelled "total women", those numbers should not be used in applying the estimation method.

Note that even if the table failed to indicate that only ever-married women were involved, the analyst should raise questions about the total female population shown, since, in a country like Bangladesh where fertility has hardly changed, it would not be expected that the number of women aged 15-19 would be smaller than the number of women aged 20-24. The very small size of age group 10-14 would also be highly suspicious and should prompt further clarification of the true meaning of the data presented.

Display 4 presents the published tabulation of the female population by age group and marital status. The numbers of women appearing in the second column, labelled "total", should be used in applying the Brass method. Note that, as expected, the number of women declines steadily with age, at least until age group 55-59 is reached.

The worksheets (displays 1 and 2) can be used to compile the information necessary for the application of the Brass method. Consider first the data on children ever born and dead. At first sight, it is unclear whether the tabulations in display 3 include the numbers of children ever born needed to apply the Brass method. The required numbers can, however, be calculated from the available data on "children at home", "children away" and "children dead". The first step is to copy the available numbers onto a reproduction of the worksheet in display 1, as shown in display 5. The next step is to calculate the missing data, children ever born, as the sum of columns 2, 4 and 5 of the worksheet in display 5. A completed worksheet, containing all the data required, is

Age group of mother	Children ever born (1) = (2) + (3) = (2) + (4) + (5)	Children dead (2) = (1) − (3) = (1) − (4) − (5)	Children surviving (3) = (4) + (5)	Children living at home (4)	Children living elsewhere (5)
Both sexes					
15-19					
20-24					
25-29					
30-34					
35-39					
40-44					
45-49					
Male					
15-19					
20-24					
25-29					
30-34					
35-39					
40-44					
45-49					
Female					
15-19					
20-24					
25-29					
30-34					
35-39					
40-44					
45-49					

Age group of women	Total number of women (1) = (2) + (3) = (4) + (5)	Ever-married women (2)	Single women (3)	Women of stated parity (4)	Women of not-stated parity (5)
15-19					
20-24					
25-29					
30-34					
35-39					
40-44					
45-49					

presented in display 6. Note that the computed numbers of children ever born shown in column 1 of display 6 are the same as those appearing in the original table (display 3) under the heading "total births". Although the data on children ever born and dead could have been copied directly from the published tabulation, it is sound practice to check the internal consistency of published data by carrying out calculations such as those illustrated in displays 5 and 6, especially when one is unsure of the meaning of certain labels ("total births" in this instance).

Turning now to the data on the total number of women by age group, recall that they should be obtained from display 4. Display 7 illustrates the compilation of those data using the worksheet shown in display 2. The worksheets in displays 6 and 7 now contain the basic data required to apply the Brass method. It is of interest, however, to explore here the consistency of the data on total number of women as derived from information contained in the original tabulations (see displays 3 and 4). Display 8 illustrates how the worksheet in display 2 may be used to compile data on the total number of women by adding the number of ever-married women copied from display 3 to the number of never-married (single) women copied from display 4. Note that the resulting total numbers of women differ, albeit slightly, from those copied directly from display 4 and shown in display 7. Such differences arise because although all ever-married women were asked about their child-bearing experience, some failed to provide the information requested and were therefore excluded from the numbers presented in display 3. Since it is suggested that *all* women, irrespective of reporting status, be used in applying the Brass method, the numbers in display 7 will be used in the examples presented in chapters IV and V.

Display 3.   Tabulation of data on children ever born and children surviving as appearing in the report on the
1974 Bangladesh Retrospective Survey of Fertility and Mortality

```
         BANGLADESH CENSUS 1974 RETROSPECTIVE SURVEY OF FERTILITY AND MORTALITY
BANGLADESH      DE FACTO

   TABLE 8 : EVER-MARRIED WOMEN BY AGE GROUP, WITH TOTAL CHILDREN EVER BORNE, NUMBER AT HOME,
             NUMBER ELSEWHERE AND NUMBER DEAD, BY SEX OF CHILDREN
```

ALL EVER-MARRIED WOMEN

AGE GROUP OF WOMEN	TOTAL WOMEN	TOTAL BIRTHS	CHILDREN AT HOME	CHILDREN AWAY	CHILDREN DEAD
TOTAL					
0–14	259 104	6 677	4 866	0	1 811
15–19	2 019 436	1 160 919	921 227	24 327	215 365
20–24	2 521 318	4 901 382	3 820 649	83 349	997 384
25–29	2 573 496	9 085 852	6 927 908	219 989	1 937 955
30–34	2 003 082	9 910 256	7 126 473	522 587	2 261 196
35–39	1 766 100	10 384 001	6 974 267	919 566	2 490 168
40–44	1 473 382	9 164 329	5 472 460	1 276 846	2 415 023
45–49	1 128 791	6 905 673	3 664 328	1 281 801	1 959 544
50–54	1 040 877	5 963 087	2 601 163	1 441 061	1 920 863
55–59	601 625	3 257 428	1 206 148	913 559	1 137 721
60+	1 631 217	8 136 608	2 102 978	2 800 615	3 233 015
N.S.	204	0	0	0	0
TOTAL	17 018 632	68 876 212	40 822 467	9 483 700	18 570 045
MALE BIRTHS ONLY					
10–14	4 111	4 112	3 109	0	1 003
15–19	501 448	597 248	469 036	11 047	117 165
20–24	1 557 199	2 507 018	1 938 220	38 921	529 877
25–29	2 106 614	4 675 978	3 545 904	82 780	1 047 294
30–34	1 792 767	5 109 487	3 780 859	124 046	1 204 582
35–39	1 635 507	5 435 726	3 925 071	176 698	1 333 957
40–44	1 369 842	4 883 599	3 323 724	268 130	1 291 745
45–49	1 047 262	3 714 957	2 393 149	291 071	1 030 737
50–54	955 899	3 211 030	1 840 032	352 615	1 018 383
55–59	545 164	1 769 751	914 419	263 461	591 871
60+	1 468 170	4 410 239	1 743 869	998 608	1 667 762
N.S.	0	0	0	0	0
TOTAL	12 983 983	36 319 145	23 877 392	2 607 377	9 834 376
FEMALE BIRTHS ONLY					
10–14	2 565	2 565	1 757	0	808
15–19	479 678	563 671	452 191	13 280	98 200
20–24	1 526 643	2 394 364	1 882 429	44 428	467 507
25–29	2 063 505	4 409 874	3 382 004	137 209	890 661
30–34	1 759 823	4 800 769	3 345 614	398 541	1 056 614
35–39	1 601 696	4 948 275	3 049 196	742 868	1 156 211
40–44	1 330 442	4 280 730	2 148 736	1 008 716	1 123 278
45–49	992 793	3 190 716	1 271 179	990 730	928 807
50–54	888 514	2 752 057	761 131	1 088 446	902 480
55–59	496 594	1 487 677	291 729	650 098	545 850
60+	1 303 670	3 726 369	359 109	1 802 007	1 565 253
N.S.	0	0	0	0	0
TOTAL	12 445 923	32 557 067	16 945 075	6 876 323	8 735 669

Source: Bangladesh, Census Commission, *Report on the 1974 Bangladesh Retrospective Survey of Fertility and Mortality* (Dacca, 1977), p. 37.

Display 4. Tabulation of the female population by age group and marital status as appearing in the report on the
1974 Bangladesh Retrospective Survey of Fertility and Mortality

```
BANGLADESH CENSUS 1974 RETROSPECTIVE SURVEY OF FERTILITY AND MORTALITY
BANGLADESH      DE FACTO

                TABLE 3.   POPULATION BY SEX, AGE GROUP, MARITAL STATUS AND NUMBER OF MARRIAGES
```

F E M A L E S

TOTAL	AGE GROUP	T O T A L	NEVER MARRIED	MARRIED	WIDOWED	DIVORCED	EVER-MARRIED NOT STATED OR EVER-MARRIED BUT PRESENT MARITAL STATUS NOT STATED
	0–4	5 490 429	5 423 807	3 121	5 961		57 540
	5–9	6 199 640	6 114 626	12 949	5 937		66 128
	10–14	4 675 449	4 353 919	256 611	4 741	15 356	44 822
	15–19	3 014 706	972 730	1 928 736	31 472	68 653	13 115
	20–24	2 653 155	121 364	2 415 049	48 242	62 586	5 914
	25–29	2 607 009	28 426	2 462 803	79 334	33 422	3 024
	30–34	2 015 663	8 365	1 871 682	115 629	15 426	4 561
	35–39	1 771 680	4 049	1 579 475	177 037	8 936	2 183
	40–44	1 479 575	3 511	1 204 957	262 790	6 764	1 553
	45–49	1 135 129	3 555	827 838	296 957	6 196	583
	50–54	1 048 558	4 183	617 085	422 448	3 665	1 177
	55–59	607 412	2 987	288 310	312 740	1 940	1 435
	60–64	697 117	6 674	227 089	460 656	1 917	781
	65–69	325 222	5 008	90 506	227 922	1 192	594
	70–74	329 326	4 156	48 907	273 108	594	2 561
	75–79	122 956	1 579	18 157	103 037	183	
	80–84	113 877	805	10 202	101 696	411	763
	85+	78 411	968	4 943	71 515	207	778
	N.S.	1 410	408	408	411		183
	TOTAL	34 366 724	17 061 120	13 868 828	3 001 633	227 448	207 695
MARRIED	0–4	8 875		3 121	5 754		
ONCE	5–9	18 132		12 766	5 366		
ONLY	10–14	273 551		253 839	4 741	14 971	
	15–19	1 952 378		1 859 246	29 878	62 864	390
	20–24	2 366 653		2 266 382	45 335	54 356	580
	25–29	2 383 749		2 282 639	72 445	28 073	592
	30–34	1 810 194		1 693 882	104 368	11 166	778
	35–39	1 580 278		1 414 313	158 431	6 759	775
	40–44	1 289 195		1 051 554	232 574	4 860	207
	45–49	1 003 347		736 408	262 710	4 229	
	50–54	923 454		547 170	373 598	2 686	
	55–59	538 306		257 196	279 945	766	399
	60–64	621 909		204 649	415 710	1 550	
	65–69	289 210		81 399	207 009	802	
	70–74	293 183		43 514	249 075	594	
	75–79	110 013		16 592	93 421		
	80–84	102 649		9 608	92 630	411	
	85+	71 890		4 736	66 947	207	
	N.S.	819		408	411		
	TOTAL	15 637 785		12 739 422	2 700 348	194 294	3 721

Source: Bangladesh, Census Commission, *Report on the 1974 Bangladesh Retrospective Survey of Fertility and Mortality* (Dacca, 1977), p. 28.

Display 5. First step in the compilation of data on children ever born and children dead for Bangladesh

Age group of mother	Children ever born (1) = (2) + (3) = (2) + (4) + (5)	Children dead (2) = (1) − (3) = (1) − (4) − (5)	Children surviving (3) = (4) + (5)	Children living at home (4)	Children living elsewhere (5)
Both sexes					
15-19		215 365		921 227	24 327
20-24		997 384		3 820 649	83 349
25-29		1 937 955		6 927 908	219 989
30-34		2 261 196		7 126 473	522 587
35-39		2 490 168		6 974 267	919 566
40-44		2 415 023		5 472 460	1 276 846
45-49		1 959 544		3 664 328	1 281 801
Male					
15-19		117 165		469 036	11 047
20-24		529 877		1 938 220	38 921
25-29		1 047 294		3 545 904	82 780
30-34		1 204 582		3 780 859	124 046
35-39		1 333 957		3 925 071	176 698
40-44		1 291 745		3 323 724	268 130
45-49		1 030 737		2 393 149	291 071
Female					
15-19		98 200		452 191	13 280
20-24		467 507		1 882 429	44 428
25-29		890 661		3 382 004	137 209
30-34		1 056 614		3 345 614	398 541
35-39		1 156 211		3 049 196	742 868
40-44		1 123 278		2 148 736	1 008 716
45-49		928 807		1 271 179	990 730

Source: Bangladesh, Census Commission, *Report on the 1974 Bangladesh Retrospective Survey of Fertility and Mortality* (Dacca, 1977), table 8, p. 37 (reproduced in display 3 above).

**Display 6. Second step in the compilation of data on children ever born
and children dead for Bangladesh**

	Age group of mother	Children ever born (1) = (2) + (3) = (2) + (4) + (5)	Children dead (2) = (1) − (3) = (1) − (4) − (5)	Children surviving (3) = (4) + (5)	Children living at home (4)	Children living elsewhere (5)
Both sexes	15-19	1 160 919	215 365		921 227	24 327
	20-24	4 901 382	997 384		3 820 649	83 349
	25-29	9 085 852	1 937 955		6 927 908	219 989
	30-34	9 910 256	2 261 196		7 126 473	522 587
	35-39	10 384 001	2 490 168		6 974 267	919 566
	40-44	9 164 329	2 415 023		5 472 460	1 276 846
	45-49	6 905 673	1 959 544		3 664 328	1 281 801
Male	15-19	597 248	117 165		469 036	11 047
	20-24	2 507 018	529 877		1 938 220	38 921
	25-29	4 675 978	1 047 294		3 545 904	82 780
	30-34	5 109 487	1 204 582		3 780 859	124 046
	35-39	5 435 726	1 333 957		3 925 071	176 698
	40-44	4 883 599	1 291 745		3 323 724	268 130
	45-49	3 714 957	1 030 737		2 393 149	291 071
Female	15-19	563 671	98 200		452 191	13 280
	20-24	2 394 364	467 507		1 882 429	44 428
	25-29	4 409 874	890 661		3 382 004	137 209
	30-34	4 800 769	1 056 614		3 345 614	398 541
	35-39	4 948 275	1 156 211		3 049 196	742 868
	40-44	4 280 780	1 123 278		2 148 736	1 008 716
	45-49	3 190 716	928 807		1 271 179	990 730

Source: Bangladesh, Census Commission, *Report on the 1974 Bangladesh Retrospective Survey of Fertility and Mortality* (Dacca, 1977), table 8, p. 37 (reproduced in display 3 above).

Display 7. Compilation of data on the total number of women by age group
for Bangladesh

Age group of women	Total number of women (1) = (2) + (3) = (4) + (5)	Ever-married women (2)	Single women (3)	Women of stated parity (4)	Women of not-stated parity (5)
15-19	3 014 706				
20-24	2 653 155				
25-29	2 607 009				
30-34	2 015 663				
35-39	1 771 680				
40-44	1 479 575				
45-49	1 135 129				

Source: Bangladesh, Census Commission, *Report on the 1974 Bangladesh Retrospective Survey of Fertility and Mortality* (Dacca, 1977), table 3, p. 28 (reproduced in display 4 above).

Display 8. Alternative compilation of data on the total number of women by age group for Bangladesh
(data rejected in the application of the Brass method)

Age group of women	Total number of women (1) = (2) + (3) = (4) + (5)	Ever-married women (2)	Single women (3)	Women of stated parity (4)	Women of not-stated parity (5)
15-19	2 992 166	2 019 436	972 730		
20-24	2 642 682	2 521 318	121 364		
25-29	2 601 922	2 573 496	28 426		
30-34	2 011 447	2 003 082	8 365		
35-39	1 770 149	1 766 100	4 049		
40-44	1 476 893	1 473 382	3 511		
45-49	1 132 346	1 128 791	3 555		

Source: Bangladesh, Census Commission, *Report on the 1974 Bangladesh Retrospective Survey of Fertility and Mortality* (Dacca, 1977), tables 3 and 8, pp. 28 and 37 (reproduced in display 4 above). Total number of women calculated as (2) + (3).

Chapter III

RATIONALE OF THE BRASS METHOD

The Brass method derives estimates of $q(x)$—the probability of dying between birth and exact age x—from the proportion of children dead among those ever borne by women in different age groups by allowing for the duration of exposure to the risk of dying. The duration of exposure is related to the age of the woman and to the timing of child-bearing. On average, the older the women, the longer ago their children would have been born and the longer the children would have been exposed to the risk of dying.

The basic relationship between the proportion of children dead by age group of mother and the probability of dying in childhood can be illustrated by a very simple example. Suppose that all women have all their children at exactly age 20. Suppose further that mortality risks are constant over time. The children of women of exact age 22 will have been exposed to the risk of dying for exactly two years, so that the proportion dead will be exactly the probability of dying by age 2, $q(2)$. Proportions dead of children ever born for women of exact ages 23 and 25 will similarly estimate $q(3)$ and $q(5)$. Note that it is the age of the women in relation to the time of child-bearing that determines the children's duration of exposure to the risk of dying and thus the relationship between the proportion dead and some $q(x)$ value.

If mortality is assumed constant, the measures of $q(2)$, $q(3)$ and $q(5)$ will be applicable to any point in time during the period preceding enumeration. Now let us consider what would happen if mortality were falling. Assume again that all women have all their children at age 20 and that we are considering women aged 22 in 1978. Then the proportion dead of the children borne by those women would estimate $q(2)$ for the cohort of children born in 1976. With mortality falling, this cohort value would be somewhat lower than the $q(2)$ in effect during 1976 (which would reflect the experience of children born during 1974, 1975 and 1976), but somewhat higher than the value for 1978 (which would reflect the experience of children born in 1976, 1977 and 1978). The $q(2)$ for the 1976 birth cohort would thus estimate the value of $q(2)$ for some time point between 1976 and 1978 (somewhat closer to 1976 than 1978 because most of the child deaths for the cohort born in 1976 would have occurred close to birth). Similarly, the proportion of children dead for women aged 23 in 1978 would estimate $q(3)$ for the cohort of children born in 1975, approximating a value of $q(3)$ for some time point close to that date. Thus, when mortality has been changing, information on the proportion of children dead can yield not only estimates of child mortality but also estimates of its trends.

The above example is, of course, greatly oversimplified. In practice, women start to bear children at different ages and have subsequent children after variable birth intervals. The proportion of children dead for women of a five-year age group represents a complex average of different probabilities of dying for varying periods. That complex average, however, depends largely on the age pattern of fertility of the women considered—which determines the distribution of children by duration of exposure to risk—and on the level and age pattern of mortality risks affecting the children.

The age pattern of child-bearing plays an important role in determining the relationship between the proportion of children dead among those borne by women of a particular age group and the children's probability of dying. To return to the simplified example above, if all women had their children at age 18 (instead of age 20) the proportion of children dead of women aged 22 would estimate the probability of dying by age 4, not age 2. Since in a life table the probability of dying by age 4, $q(4)$, must be greater than the probability of dying by age 2, $q(2)$, a given proportion of children dead for women aged 22 would indicate lower mortality risks in an early-fertility population than in a late-fertility population. Put another way, the children of women of a given age in an early-fertility population would, on average, have been born longer ago and would therefore have been exposed longer to the risks of dying than children of women of the same age in a late-child-bearing population. It is for this reason that fertility patterns must be taken into account in converting proportions of children dead into probabilities of dying.

The Brass method makes allowance for the pattern of fertility in a population by considering the lifetime fertility of women in different age groups. The measure of lifetime fertility used is called average parity, which is defined as the average number of children ever born per woman of a given age group. (It is calculated by dividing the total number of children ever borne by women of a given age group by the total number of women in that age group.)

If fertility has been constant, the average parity of women now aged, say, 15 to 19 will be the same as the average parity five years ago of women who are now aged 20 to 24. Thus, the current distribution of average parities by age group can be used as an indicator of the shape of the lifetime fertility distribution that needs to be considered in converting proportions of children dead into probabilities of dying in childhood. Specifically, using $P(1)$, $P(2)$ and $P(3)$ to denote the average parities of women in age groups 15-19, 20-24 and 25-29, respectively, allowance for the pattern of fertility is made by using the parity ratios $P(1)/P(2)$ and $P(2)/P(3)$. Note that, because parity ratios are used, the actual level of fertility does not matter, only its age pattern. For example, the greater $P(1)/P(2)$, the earlier the pattern of child-bearing.

DERIVATION OF THE METHOD

The actual derivation of a Brass-type estimation procedure involves the use of simulation to generate proportions of children dead, the probabilities of dying that they are related to, and the parity ratios $P(1)/P(2)$ and $P(2)/P(3)$ that link them. Regression analysis is used to derive estimation equations, which make the application of the procedure straightforward.

It is worth nothing that there are several versions of the Brass method. They differ mostly in the type of models used to simulate the quantities of interest. The two versions described in this *Guide* are those proposed by Trussell (1975) and by Palloni and Heligman (1986). They differ mainly in that the former uses the Coale-Demeny regional model life tables to simulate mortality, while the latter uses the United Nations model life tables for developing countries. Both versions are presented here in order to provide the analyst with a wide choice of possible mortality models.

Table 3 indicates how all Brass-type estimation procedures link estimated $q(x)$ values with the observed proportions of children dead by age of mother, denoted by $D(i)$. As indicated in the table, an estimate of the probability of dying by age 1, $q(1)$, can be derived from the proportion of children dead reported by women aged 15-19, $D(1)$; the probability of dying by age 2, $q(2)$, can be obtained from the proportion of children dead for women aged 20-24, $D(2)$, and so on.

TABLE 3. CORRESPONDENCE BETWEEN OBSERVED PROPORTIONS OF CHILDREN DEAD BY AGE GROUP OF MOTHER AND ESTIMATED PROBABILITIES OF DYING

Age group of mother	Age group index i	Proportion of children dead $D(i)$	Estimated probability of dying by age x $q(x)$
15-19	1	$D(1)$	$q(1)$
20-24	2	$D(2)$	$q(2)$
25-29	3	$D(3)$	$q(3)$
30-34	4	$D(4)$	$q(5)$
35-39	5	$D(5)$	$q(10)$
40-44	6	$D(6)$	$q(15)$
45-49	7	$D(7)$	$q(20)$

ESTIMATING TIME TRENDS OF MORTALITY

The method originally developed by Brass assumed that mortality was constant, so that cohort and period probabilities of dying were identical. That assumption was later relaxed through the work of Feeney (1980), Coale and Trussell (1978) and others. Those authors showed that if the rate of change of mortality over time was approximately constant, the reference date of each $q(x)$ could be estimated by making allowance for the age pattern of fertility by means of the $P(1)/P(2)$ and $P(2)/P(3)$ ratios.

Since the measurement of child mortality trends is a major objective of this *Guide*, the use of the Brass method to detect or quantify changes in such trends resulting from programme activities requires further discussion. The procedure for estimating the reference dates of $q(x)$ values assumes that mortality has been changing steadily over time. A programme that speeds mortality decline will invalidate this assumption. Such a change in trend will have a greater effect on the proportions of children dead of younger women—a higher proportion of whose children will have been exposed to the recently lower mortality risks—than on the proportions of children dead of older women. It will also have some effect on such proportions for women of any age having significant numbers of recent births. Consequently, the Brass method will smooth out any sharp change in trend, transforming it into a gradually accelerating decline and thus making it harder to associate a decline with programme activities.

It should also be noted that the Brass method is unlikely to indicate any change in trend until at least two years after the change occurs. This lag arises from the observation, discussed in greater detail below, that mortality estimates based on reports of women aged 15-19—which reflect the most recent mortality—are generally unreliable.

LIMITATIONS OF THE BRASS METHOD ASSOCIATED
WITH ITS SIMPLIFYING ASSUMPTIONS

The Brass method is based on certain simplifying assumptions that may not be entirely satisfied in practice and that have implications for the interpretation of the estimates obtained.

The Brass method assumes that the mortality risks of children of women who do not report their child-bearing experience are the same as those of children whose mothers do. Aside from the problem of women who do not provide information, women may have moved away from the survey area before being interviewed or may have died. Thus, the estimates obtained assume, among other things, that the survivorship of children is independent of that of their mothers.

The method also assumes that fertility has remained constant during the 30 or 35 years preceding the survey or census. If fertility has been changing, the parity ratios will be affected, and the allowance made for the age pattern of child-bearing will not be correct. In particular, if fertility has been declining, the parity ratios will be too low, indicating a later age pattern of fertility than the actual one and leading to an overestimate of child mortality.

Perhaps the most basic assumption of the method is that the reported proportions of children dead are correct.

23

If some of the children that have died are reported as being alive or if dead children are omitted to a greater extent than living children, the mortality estimates obtained will be too low. If, as is generally the case, omissions and other errors are more prevalent among older than younger women, certain patterns in the data may indicate that errors have occurred. For example, the mortality estimates based on reports of women aged 40 and over may fail to increase with age of mother at the same pace as those based on the reports of younger women. Furthermore, the average parities of women aged 35 and over may not increase with age (or may actually decrease at older ages), indicating possible omissions of dead children.

Lastly, the Brass method assumes that mortality risks among children depend solely on their age and not on other factors, such as age of mother or birth order. If, for example, the mortality risks of children borne by young mothers (under age 20) were higher than average, then the proportion of children dead reported by women aged 15-19 would be too high and therefore would overestimate overall mortality levels. In addition, the estimates derived from data on women aged 20-24 might also be upwardly biased, since a significant proportion of the children reported by women aged 20-24 would have been born when the women were 15-19. By age group 25-29, however, a high proportion of all children would have been borne by mothers aged 20 and over, so that the effect of the abnormally high risks experienced by children of young mothers on the estimate of $q(5)$ would be small.

In practice, child mortality estimates based on reports of women aged 15-19 and, to a lesser extent, on those of women aged 20-24 are generally unreliable, often being higher than estimates based on reports of older women. The detailed example presented in the next chapter illustrates this effect and shows why the Brass method is not capable of providing reliable estimates of very recent mortality conditions (those prevalent during the two or even three years preceding interview).

Chapter IV

TRUSSELL VERSION OF THE BRASS METHOD

This version of the Brass method was developed during the late 1970s by T. J. Trussell (United Nations, 1983b, chap. III). It is based on the Coale-Demeny model life tables, and it has the advantage over earlier versions of producing estimates both of probabilities of dying from birth to different ages in childhood and of the time point to which each probability refers.

The following section presents step by step the computational procedure to be followed in applying the Trussell version. The case of Bangladesh is then used to give a detailed example of its application.

COMPUTATIONAL PROCEDURE

Step 1. *Calculation of average parity per woman*

Average parity is the average number of children ever borne by women in a given five-year age group. It is calculated as

$$P(i) = \frac{CEB(i)}{FP(i)} \qquad (4.1)$$

where $P(i)$ is the average parity of women of age group i, $CEB(i)$ is the total number of children ever borne by these women, and $FP(i)$ is the total number of women in the age group irrespective of their marital or reporting status. Although parity values are needed only for age groups 15-19, 20-24 and 25-29—$P(1)$, $P(2)$ and $P(3)$, respectively—it is worth calculating the whole set up to age group 45-49 in order to check the quality of the basic data. Note that the denominator, $FP(i)$, should include even those women who did not respond to the questions on children ever born (those of not-stated parity). Their inclusion is based on the assumption that they are childless, an assumption supported by evidence from a large number of surveys showing that the vast majority of younger women reported as being of not-stated parity are, in fact, childless.

Step 2. *Calculation of the proportions dead among children ever born*

The proportion of children dead is given simply by the ratio of the total number of dead children to the total number of children ever born (including those who have died) for each age group. Thus,

$$D(i) = \frac{CD(i)}{CEB(i)} \qquad (4.2)$$

where $D(i)$ is the proportion of children dead for women of age group i, $CD(i)$ is the number of children dead reported by those women, and $CEB(i)$ is the total number of children ever borne by those women.

Step 3. *Calculation of the multipliers, k(i)*

The basic estimation equation for the Trussell method is

$$q(x) = k(i) D(i) \qquad (4.3)$$

where

$$k(i) = a(i) + b(i) \frac{P(1)}{P(2)} + c(i) \frac{P(2)}{P(3)} \qquad (4.4)$$

Thus, the mortality measure $q(x)$, the probability of dying by exact age x, is related to the proportion dead $D(i)$ by a multiplying factor $k(i)$ that is determined by the parity ratios $P(1)/P(2)$ and $P(2)/P(3)$ and three coefficients $a(i)$, $b(i)$ and $c(i)$. These coefficients were estimated by regression analysis of simulated model cases. Table 4 shows the coefficients for the seven age groups of women, from ages 15-19 through ages 45-49 $(i = 1, \ldots, 7)$, and for the four regional families of the Coale-Demeny model life tables.

Step 4. *Calculation of the probabilities of dying by age x, q(x)*

Once $D(i)$ and $k(i)$ have been calculated for each age group i, estimates of $q(x)$ are obtained simply as their product, as already indicated in equation 4.3:

$$q(x) = k(i)D(i)$$

Step 5. *Calculation of the reference dates for q(x), t(i)*

As explained earlier, under conditions of steady mortality change over time, a reference time, $t(i)$, can be estimated for each $q(x)$ estimated in step 4. This reference time is expressed in terms of number of years before the survey or census and is estimated through the use of coefficients applied to parity ratios. As before, the coefficients were estimated by regression analysis of simulated model cases. The estimating equation is

$$t(i) = e(i) + f(i) \frac{P(1)}{P(2)} + g(i) \frac{P(2)}{P(3)} \qquad (4.5)$$

Table 5 shows the coefficients $e(i)$, $f(i)$ and $g(i)$ for use in equation 4.5 for each age group of women and for each of the four Coale-Demeny model-life-table families.

Once values of $t(i)$ are obtained, they can be converted into actual dates by subtracting them from the reference date of the survey or census expressed in decimal terms, as illustrated in the detailed example below.

Step 6. *Conversion to a common index*

Steps 4 and 5 provide estimates of $q(x)$ for ages x of 1, 2, 3, 5, 10, 15 and 20 and of $t(i)$, the number of years

25

TABLE 4. COEFFICIENTS FOR THE ESTIMATION OF CHILD-MORTALITY MULTIPLIERS, $k(i)$, TRUSSELL VERSION OF THE BRASS METHOD, USING THE COALE-DEMENY MORTALITY MODELS

Model	Age group of mother (1)	Age group Index i (2)	Age x of children (3)	Coefficients $a(i)$ (4)	$b(i)$ (5)	$c(i)$ (6)
North......................	15-19	1	1	1.1119	−2.9287	0.8507
	20-24	2	2	1.2390	−0.6865	−0.2745
	25-29	3	3	1.1884	0.0421	−0.5156
	30-34	4	5	1.2046	0.3037	−0.5656
	35-39	5	10	1.2586	0.4236	−0.5898
	40-44	6	15	1.2240	0.4222	−0.5456
	45-49	7	20	1.1772	0.3486	−0.4624
South	15-19	1	1	1.0819	−3.0005	0.8689
	20-24	2	2	1.2846	−0.6181	−0.3024
	25-29	3	3	1.2223	0.0851	−0.4704
	30-34	4	5	1.1905	0.2631	−0.4487
	35-39	5	10	1.1911	0.3152	−0.4291
	40-44	6	15	1.1564	0.3017	−0.3958
	45-49	7	20	1.1307	0.2596	−0.3538
East......................	15-19	1	1	1.1461	−2.2536	0.6259
	20-24	2	2	1.2231	−0.4301	−0.2245
	25-29	3	3	1.1593	0.0581	−0.3479
	30-34	4	5	1.1404	0.1991	−0.3487
	35-39	5	10	1.1540	0.2511	−0.3506
	40-44	6	15	1.1336	0.2556	−0.3428
	45-49	7	20	1.1201	0.2362	−0.3268
West......................	15-19	1	1	1.1415	−2.7070	0.7663
	20-24	2	2	1.2563	−0.5381	−0.2637
	25-29	3	3	1.1851	0.0633	−0.4177
	30-34	4	5	1.1720	0.2341	−0.4272
	35-39	5	10	1.1865	0.3080	−0.4452
	40-44	6	15	1.1746	0.3314	−0.4537
	45-49	7	20	1.1639	0.3190	−0.4435

Estimation equations:

$$k(i) = a(i) + b(i)\frac{P(1)}{P(2)} + c(i)\frac{P(2)}{P(3)}$$

$$q(x) = k(i)\, D(i)$$

Source: *Manual X: Indirect Techniques for Demographic Estimation*, Population Studies, No. 81 (United Nations publication, Sales No. E.83.XIII.2), p. 77.

before the survey to which each estimate applies. In order to analyse trends and facilitate comparison both within and between data sets, each estimated $q(x)$ is converted to a single measure. Although any index from the model-life-table family can be used for that purpose, it is suggested that a measure of mortality in childhood that is not particularly sensitive to the pattern of mortality be selected. The common index recommended is the probability of dying by age 5, $q(5)$, also called under-five mortality. The use of infant mortality as the common index is not recommended because, as will be seen, the estimates of $q(1)$ obtained from the conversion are very sensitive to the mortality pattern underlying the different models.

The $q(x)$ values corresponding to the model-life-table family being considered can be used to carry out the required conversions. The tables in annex I contain the necessary values of $q(x)$ ordered by mortality level and expectation of life for each of the Coale-Demeny families of model life tables (see chap. I) and for males, females and both sexes separately. The actual conversion is carried out by linear interpolation between tabulated values, as explained below.

Suppose that an estimated value of $q(x)$, denoted by $q^e(x)$, is to be converted to the corresponding $q^c(5)$ where, of course, $x \neq 5$. For a given model-life-table family and sex, it is first necessary to identify the mortality levels with $q(x)$ values that enclose the estimated value, $q^e(x)$. Thus, the task is to identify in the appropriate table of annex I levels j and $j + 1$ such that

$$q^j(x) > q^e(x) > q^{j+1}(x) \tag{4.6}$$

where $q^j(x)$ and $q^{j+1}(x)$ are the model values of $q(x)$ for levels j and $j + 1$, respectively, and $q^e(x)$ is the estimated value. Then, the desired common index $q^c(5)$ is given by

$$q^c(5) = (1.0 - h)\, q^j(5) + h\, q^{j+1}(5) \tag{4.7}$$

where h is the interpolation factor calculated in the following way:

26

Model	Age group of mother (1)	Age group Index i (2)	Estimated $q(x)$ (3)	Coefficients $e(i)$ (4)	$f(i)$ (5)	$g(i)$ (6)
North	15-19	1	$q(1)$	1.0921	5.4732	− 1.9672
	20-24	2	$q(2)$	1.3207	5.3751	0.2133
	25-29	3	$q(3)$	1.5996	2.6268	4.3701
	30-34	4	$q(5)$	2.0779	− 1.7908	9.4126
	35-39	5	$q(10)$	2.7705	− 7.3403	14.9352
	40-44	6	$q(15)$	4.1520	− 12.2448	19.2349
	45-49	7	$q(20)$	6.9650	− 13.9160	19.9542
South	15-19	1	$q(1)$	1.0900	5.4443	− 1.9721
	20-24	2	$q(2)$	1.3079	5.5568	0.2021
	25-29	3	$q(3)$	1.5173	2.6755	4.7471
	30-34	4	$q(5)$	1.9399	− 2.2739	10.3876
	35-39	5	$q(10)$	2.6157	− 8.4819	16.5153
	40-44	6	$q(15)$	4.0794	− 13.8308	21.1866
	45-49	7	$q(20)$	7.1796	− 15.3880	21.7892
East	15-19	1	$q(1)$	1.0959	5.5864	− 1.9949
	20-24	2	$q(2)$	1.2921	5.5897	0.3631
	25-29	3	$q(3)$	1.5021	2.4692	5.0927
	30-34	4	$q(5)$	1.9347	− 2.6419	10.8533
	35-39	5	$q(10)$	2.6197	− 8.9693	17.0981
	40-44	6	$q(15)$	4.1317	− 14.3550	21.8247
	45-49	7	$q(20)$	7.3657	− 15.8083	22.3005
West	15-19	1	$q(1)$	1.0970	5.5628	− 1.9956
	20-24	2	$q(2)$	1.3062	5.5677	0.2962
	25-29	3	$q(3)$	1.5305	2.5528	4.8962
	30-34	4	$q(5)$	1.9991	− 2.4261	10.4282
	35-39	5	$q(10)$	2.7632	− 8.4065	16.1787
	40-44	6	$q(15)$	4.3468	− 13.2436	20.1990
	45-49	7	$q(20)$	7.5242	− 14.2013	20.0162

Estimation equation:

$$t(i) = e(i) + f(i)\frac{P(1)}{P(2)} + g(i)\frac{P(2)}{P(3)}$$

Source: *Manual X: Indirect Techniques for Demographic Estimation*, Population Studies, No. 81 (United Nations publication, Sales No. E.83.XIII.2), p. 78.

[a] Number of years prior to the survey.

$$h = \frac{q^e(x) - q^j(x)}{q^{j+1}(x) - q^j(x)} \qquad (4.8)$$

If the data on children ever born and children dead are for both sexes combined, the model $q^j(x)$ values should be taken from the tables for both sexes combined in annex I. If, however, the data are for male and female children separately, the estimated values of $q(x)$ will be sex-specific, and the conversion to a common index should use the model $q^j(x)$ values from the tables for the relevant sex, also presented in annex I.

Step 7. *Interpretation and analysis of results*

Once seven estimates (one for each age group i of women) of the selected common index—$q^c(5)$ as suggested above—have been obtained, it is recommended that they be plotted against time. As noted in step 5, the $t(i)$ values can be converted into reference dates by subtracting them from the survey or census reference date (or the approximate midpoint of the field-work), and the $q^c(5)$ estimates can then be plotted against the resulting dates. Graphical presentation of the results is essential to assess the consistency and general trend of the estimates, as the example below illustrates.

A DETAILED EXAMPLE

Compilation of the data required

The data gathered by the 1974 Bangladesh Retrospective Survey of Fertility and Mortality will be used to illustrate the application of the Trussell version of the Brass method. In chapter II, the data necessary to apply the method were compiled in displays 6 and 7 (they are shown here again for convenience). Since the basic data are available by sex, they will be used to check the internal consistency of the information on children ever born.

Table 6 illustrates how the sex ratio at birth is calculated from the data on children ever born for different age groups of mother by dividing the number of male children by the number of female children ever born. The sex ratio at birth is biologically determined and varies relatively little, ranging usually between 1.03 and 1.08 male births per female birth. Table 6 shows that up

Display 6. Second step in the compilation of data on children ever born
and children dead for Bangladesh

	Age group of mother	Children ever born (1) = (2) + (3) = (2) + (4) + (5)	Children dead (2) = (1) − (3) = (1) − (4) − (5)	Children surviving (3) = (4) + (5)	Children living at home (4)	Children living elsewhere (5)
Both sexes	15-19	1 160 919	215 365		921 227	24 327
	20-24	4 901 382	997 384		3 820 649	83 349
	25-29	9 085 852	1 937 955		6 927 908	219 989
	30-34	9 910 256	2 261 196		7 126 473	522 587
	35-39	10 384 001	2 490 168		6 974 267	919 566
	40-44	9 164 329	2 415 023		5 472 460	1 276 846
	45-49	6 905 673	1 959 544		3 664 328	1 281 801
Male	15-19	597 248	117 165		469 036	11 047
	20-24	2 507 018	529 877		1 938 220	38 921
	25-29	4 675 978	1 047 294		3 545 904	82 780
	30-34	5 109 487	1 204 582		3 780 859	124 046
	35-39	5 435 726	1 333 957		3 925 071	176 698
	40-44	4 883 599	1 291 745		3 323 724	268 130
	45-49	3 714 957	1 030 737		2 393 149	291 071
Female	15-19	563 671	98 200		452 191	13 280
	20-24	2 394 364	467 507		1 882 429	44 428
	25-29	4 409 874	890 661		3 382 004	137 209
	30-34	4 800 769	1 056 614		3 345 614	398 541
	35-39	4 948 275	1 156 211		3 049 196	742 868
	40-44	4 280 730	1 123 278		2 148 736	1 008 716
	45-49	3 190 716	928 807		1 271 179	990 730

Source: Bangladesh, Census Commission, *Report on the 1974 Bangladesh Retrospective Survey of Fertility and Mortality* (Dacca, 1977), table 8, p. 37 (reproduced in display 3 above).

Display 7. Compilation of data on the total number of women
by age group for Bangladesh

Age group of women	Total number of women (1) = (2) + (3) = (4) + (5)	Ever-married women (2)	Single women (3)	Women of stated parity (4)	Women of not-stated parity (5)
15-19	3 014 706				
20-24	2 653 155				
25-29	2 607 009				
30-34	2 015 663				
35-39	1 771 680				
40-44	1 479 575				
45-49	1 135 129				

Source: Bangladesh, Census Commission, *Report on the 1974 Bangladesh Retrospective Survey of Fertility and Mortality* (Dacca, 1977), table 3, p. 28 (reproduced in display 4 above).

to age group 30-34 the reported numbers of male and female children ever born yield sex ratios at birth within the expected range. Over age 35, however, the sex ratios at birth are too high, implying that too many males were reported relative to females. Such a pattern suggests that the data on children ever born corresponding to older women (aged 35 and over) are probably affected by the omission of female children, though misreporting of the children's sex also could give rise to the same pattern.

TABLE 6. CALCULATION OF THE SEX RATIO AT BIRTH FROM DATA ON CHILDREN EVER BORN, CLASSIFIED BY SEX, FROM THE 1974 BANGLADESH RETROSPECTIVE SURVEY

Age group of mother (1)	Male children ever born (2)	Female children ever born (3)	Sex ratio at birth (4) = (2)/(3)
15-19	597 248	563 671	1.060
20-24	2 507 018	2 394 364	1.047
25-29	4 675 978	4 409 874	1.060
30-34	5 109 487	4 800 769	1.064
35-39	5 435 726	4 948 275	1.099
40-44	4 883 599	4 280 730	1.141
45-49	3 714 957	3 190 716	1.164

Computational procedure

Step 1. *Calculation of average parity per woman*

To apply the method, average parities are used to calculate the parity ratios $P(1)/P(2)$ and $P(2)/P(3)$. Thus, parities need to be calculated only for women aged 15-19, 20-24 and 25-29. However, it is good practice to calculate parities for all seven age groups of women, because they can reveal problems with the basic data.

In this example mortality will be estimated for both sexes combined, so parities should be calculated using the data on children ever born of both sexes appearing in the top panel of display 6. Each parity $P(i)$ will therefore be obtained by dividing those numbers by the total number of women shown in display 7, age group by age group. Thus, for women aged 25-29 $(i=3)$,

$$P(3) = \frac{9,085,852}{2,607,009} = 3.4852$$

Column 3 of table 7 shows the complete set of average parities by age group. Notice that they do not increase steadily with age. In particular, the average parity for women aged 45-49 is lower than that for women aged 40-44, which is not consistent with the existence of constant fertility in the past. The increase in the average parity from age group 35-39 to age group 40-44 also seems too small. Such a pattern of change with age in the average parities, coupled with the high sex ratios at birth noticed among the children of older women, strongly suggests that there are omission errors in their reports of lifetime fertility. Because dead children are more likely to be omitted than live ones, evidence of omission requires that the resulting mortality estimates be interpreted with caution.

Step 2. *Calculation of the proportions dead among children ever born*

The proportions dead, denoted by $D(i)$, are calculated as the ratios of the number of children dead to the number of children ever borne by women of each age group i. Such ratios are obtained in this case by dividing the entries in column 2 of display 6 by those of column 1

TABLE 7. APPLICATION OF THE TRUSSELL VERSION OF THE BRASS METHOD TO DATA ON BOTH SEXES FROM THE 1974 BANGLADESH RETROSPECTIVE SURVEY

Age group of mother (1)	Age group index (i) (2)	Average parity P(i) (3)	Proportion dead D(i) (4)	Multiplier k(i) (5)	Age x (6)	Probability of dying by age x, q(x) (7)	Time reference t(i) (8)	Reference date (9)	Common index $q^c(5)$ (10)
15-19	1	0.3851	.1855	0.9169	1	.170	1.2	1973.1	.294
20-24	2	1.8474	.2035	0.9954	2	.203	2.6	1971.7	.248
25-29	3	3.4852	.2133	0.9907	3	.211	4.6	1969.7	.230
30-34	4	4.9166	.2282	1.0075	5	.230	7.0	1967.3	.230
35-39	5	5.8611	.2398	1.0294	10	.247	9.6	1964.7	.229
40-44	6	6.1940	.2635	1.0095	15	.266	12.4	1961.9	.237
45-49	7	6.0836	.2838	0.9973	20	.283	15.5	1958.8	.239

$P(1)/P(2) = .2085$
$P(2)/P(3) = .5301$

Multipliers based on South model.
Sex ratio at birth = 1.05

for both sexes combined. Thus, for women aged 25-29 and $i = 3$,

$$D(3) = \frac{1,937,955}{9,085,852} = .2133$$

Results for all age groups, $i = 1, \ldots, 7$, are shown in column 4 of table 7.

Step 3. *Calculation of the multipliers, k(i)*

The multipliers $k(i)$ are calculated for each age group i using a set of coefficients from table 4 and the ratios of average parities $P(1)/P(2)$ and $P(2)/P(3)$. Those ratios can be computed from column 3 of table 7:

$$\frac{P(1)}{P(2)} = \frac{.3851}{1.8474} = .2085$$

$$\frac{P(2)}{P(3)} = \frac{1.8474}{3.4852} = .5301$$

The regression coefficients $a(i)$, $b(i)$ and $c(i)$ in table 4 are specified for each family of the Coale-Demeny model life tables. The South family has been selected for use in this example, so that the coefficients in the second panel of table 4 will be used. For each age group i, $k(i)$ is computed using equation 4.4. Thus, for age group 3, in which women are aged 25-29,

$$k(3) = 1.2223 + (.0851)(.2085) + (-.4704)(.5301)$$
$$= .9907$$

The complete set of $k(i)$ values is shown in column 5 of table 7.

Step 4. *Calculation of the probabilities of dying by age x, q(x)*

The $q(x)$ is computed for each age group i by multiplying the proportion of children dead, $D(i)$, by the multiplier $k(i)$. The correspondence between x values and i values is shown in table 3. Hence, for age group 3, in which women are aged 25-29, x is equal to 3, and $q(3)$ is given as

$$q(3) = k(3) D(3) = (.9907)(.2133) = .2110$$

indicating a probability of dying by age 3 of 21.1 per cent. The probabilities of dying, $q(x)$, for all seven age groups of mother are shown in column 7 of table 7.

Step 5. *Calculation of the reference dates for* q(x), t(i)

The time reference $t(i)$ for each estimated $q(x)$ in number of years before the survey is calculated according to equation 4.5 from the two parity ratios $P(1)/P(2)$ and $P(2)/P(3)$ and the three coefficients $e(i)$, $g(i)$ and $h(i)$ that correspond to the model-life-table pattern selected.

In the case of Bangladesh, the coefficients shown in the second panel of table 5, corresponding to the South model, will be used. Considering once more age group 3 (women aged 25-29), one gets

$$t(3) = 1.5173 + (2.6755)(.2085) + (4.7471)(.5301)$$
$$= 4.59$$

That is, under conditions of steady mortality decline, the estimate of $q(3)$ obtained from the proportion of children dead among those ever borne by women aged 25-29 would refer to a period nearly four and a half years before the survey. Since, in this particular case, the survey's field-work was carried out mostly during April 1974, the survey's reference date can be taken to be 1974.3—15 April corresponds to day number 105 in the year, which, divided by the total number of days in a year, is $105/365 = 0.29$, a figure that is rounded to 0.3 in decimal terms. Hence, the reference date for the estimated $q(3)$ is

$$1974.3 - 4.6 = 1969.7$$

or towards the end of the calendar year 1969. The other values of $t(i)$ and the reference dates calculated from them are shown in columns 8 and 9 of table 7.

Step 6. *Conversion to a common index*

In order to study trends in child mortality, the $q(x)$ values obtained in step 4 need to be converted to a common index. Under-five mortality, $q(5)$, will be used here as the common index. The conversion is carried out by interpolating between the $q(x)$ values of the model life tables presented in annex I. The table used for interpolation—table A.I.10—is that for model South and both sexes combined (the values it displays were derived assuming a sex ratio at birth of 1.05 male births per female birth).

As an example, consider the conversion of the estimated $q^e(3)$ to a $q^c(5)$ according to model South.

The estimated value of $q^e(3)$ is .211. According to table A.I.10, this value falls between the $q(3)$ of level 12, $q^{12}(3) = .22564$, whose $q^{12}(5)$ equivalent is .24592, and that of level 13, $q^{13}(3) = .20640$, whose $q^{13}(5)$ equivalent is .22430. Substituting the $q^j(3)$ and $q^e(3)$ values in equation 4.8 to find h, the interpolation factor, one obtains

$$h = \frac{.21100 - .22564}{.20604 - .22564} = .7469$$

The $q^c(5)$ equivalent for the estimated $q^e(3) = .211$ is then derived using equation 4.7 as follows:

$$q^c(5) = (1.0 - .7469)(.24592) + (.7469)(.22430)$$
$$= .230$$

That is, in the South model life tables, the $q^c(5)$ corresponding to a $q^e(3)$ of .211 is .230. The complete set of $q^c(5)$ values equivalent to the estimated $q(x)$ values is shown in column 10 of table 7.

Step 7. *Interpretation and analysis of results*

Once the values of the common index $q^c(5)$ have been derived for all age groups of women, they can be plotted against the reference date for each estimate, as shown in figure 7. That figure shows clearly that the estimated $q^c(5)$ values are fairly similar for most of the period 1959-1970 and that they increase markedly after 1970. Therefore, taken at face value, those estimates imply that in Bangladesh mortality in childhood increased during the early 1970s after varying within a narrow range during the preceding decade. Such an interpretation is not correct. As figure 7 indicates, the estimates referring to recent periods (1972 onwards) are those derived from the reports of younger women (age groups 20-24 and 15-19) and hence reflect the higher than average risks of dying to which the children of those women are subject. Furthermore, given the evidence available on the existence of omissions of children ever born in the reports of older women (aged 35 and over), it is likely that the estimates referring to periods furthest in the past (1959-1965 or thereabouts) may be biased downward. As a result of both biases, the curve displayed in figure 7 probably fails to reflect the actual trend of under-five mortality, $q(5)$, in Bangladesh. Unfortunately, the true trend cannot be derived with certainty from the data available. However, it can be established with a high degree of confidence that during the 1965-1970 period under-five mortality in Bangladesh was approximately .230, that is, during the late 1960s slightly more than one out of every five children born would die before reaching the fifth birthday.

Figure 7. Under-five mortality, $q(5)$, for both sexes in Bangladesh, estimated
using model South and the Trussell version of the Brass method

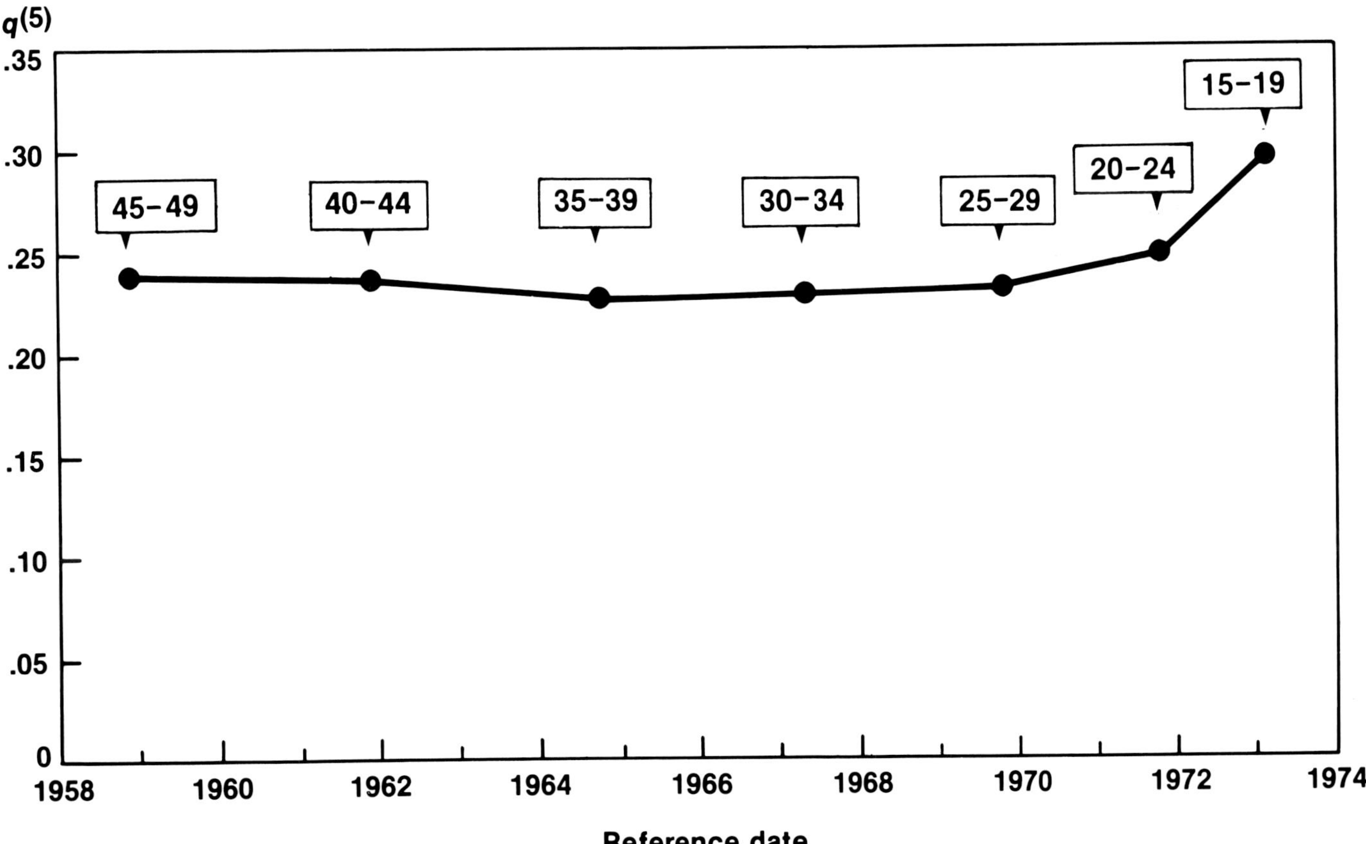

Another conclusion that can be drawn from the estimates available so far is that mortality in childhood in Bangladesh probably did not change much during the 1960s. Of course, given the downward bias that probably affects earlier estimates, such an assertion cannot be made with absolute certainty. As the next section will show, the availability of further evidence may modify this preliminary conclusion.

Estimates of mortality in childhood by sex

As shown in display 6, the data on children ever born and surviving for Bangladesh are available by sex of child. It is therefore possible to estimate mortality by sex. To estimate male mortality, for instance, the procedure to be followed is essentially the same as that described above, except that parities and the proportions dead are calculated only on the basis of male children. In algebraic terms, letting the subindex m denote male, in step 1 equation 4.1 becomes

$$P_m(i) = \frac{CEB_m(i)}{FP(i)} \qquad (4.9)$$

and in step 2 equation 4.2 becomes

$$D_m(i) = \frac{CD_m(i)}{CEB_m(i)} \qquad (4.10)$$

That is, the average parities are calculated by dividing the number of male children ever born by the total female population, as in equation 4.9, and the proportion of male children dead, $D_m(i)$, for each age group is calculated by dividing the number of male children dead by the number of male children ever born. Steps 3 to 7 are then carried out as indicated in the computational procedure. Female mortality in childhood is estimated in the same way, substituting female children ever born and dead instead of the corresponding male children.

Tables 8 and 9 show the results of applying the Trussell version of the Brass method to the Bangladesh data classified by sex. Figure 8 plots the estimated under-five mortality, $q(5)$, for males and females. Note that for most age groups of mother the male estimates of $q(5)$ are higher than those for females. Since higher male than female mortality is the rule in most countries, the 1961-1974 estimates for Bangladesh seem acceptable. However, the reversal of the relationship between male and female mortality for the estimates derived from age group 45-49 is suspect, being in all probability caused by errors in the basic data rather than by the actual reversal of mortality differentials by sex. For that reason, the estimates derived from the reports of women aged 45-49 should be disregarded, even when they refer to both sexes combined.

TABLE 8. APPLICATION OF THE TRUSSELL VERSION OF THE BRASS METHOD TO DATA ON MALES FROM THE 1974 BANGLADESH RETROSPECTIVE SURVEY

Age group of mother (1)	Age group index (i) (2)	Average parity $P_m(i)$ (3)	Proportion dead $D_m(i)$ (4)	Multiplier $k(i)$ (5)	Age x (6)	Probability of dying by age x, $q_m(x)$ (7)	Time reference $t(i)$ (8)	Reference date (9)	Common index $q_m^c(5)$ (10)
15-19	1	0.1981	.1962	0.9104	1	.179	1.2	1973.1	.301
20-24	2	0.9449	.2114	0.9957	2	.210	2.6	1971.7	.256
25-29	3	1.7936	.2240	0.9923	3	.222	4.6	1969.7	.241
30-34	4	2.5349	.2358	1.0093	5	.238	6.9	1967.4	.238
35-39	5	3.0681	.2454	1.0312	10	.253	9.5	1964.8	.236
40-44	6	3.3007	.2645	1.0112	15	.268	12.3	1962.0	.240
45-49	7	3.2727	.2775	0.9988	20	.277	15.4	1958.9	.236

$P_m(1)/P_m(2) = .2097$
$P_m(2)/P_m(3) = .5268$
Multipliers based on South model.

TABLE 9. APPLICATION OF THE TRUSSELL VERSION OF THE BRASS METHOD TO DATA ON FEMALES FROM THE 1974 BANGLADESH RETROSPECTIVE SURVEY

Age group of mother (1)	Age group index (i) (2)	Average parity $P_f(i)$ (3)	Proportion dead $D_f(i)$ (4)	Multiplier $k(i)$ (5)	Age x (6)	Probability of dying by age x, $q_f(x)$ (7)	Time reference $t(i)$ (8)	Reference date (9)	Common index $q_f^c(5)$ (10)
15-19	1	0.1897	.1742	0.9238	1	.161	1.2	1973.1	.286
20-24	2	0.9025	.1953	0.9952	2	.194	2.6	1971.7	.240
25-29	3	1.6916	.2020	0.9890	3	.200	4.6	1969.7	.218
30-34	4	2.3817	.2201	1.0056	5	.221	7.0	1967.3	.221
35-39	5	2.7930	.2337	1.0275	10	.240	9.7	1964.6	.222
40-44	6	2.8932	.2624	1.0078	15	.264	12.5	1961.8	.234
45-49	7	2.8109	.2911	0.9957	20	.290	15.6	1958.7	.243

$P_f(1)/P_f(2) = .2072$
$P_f(2)/P_f(3) = .5335$
Multipliers based on South model.

Figure 8. Under-five mortality, $q(5)$, for males and females in Bangladesh, estimated using model South and the Trussell version of the Brass method

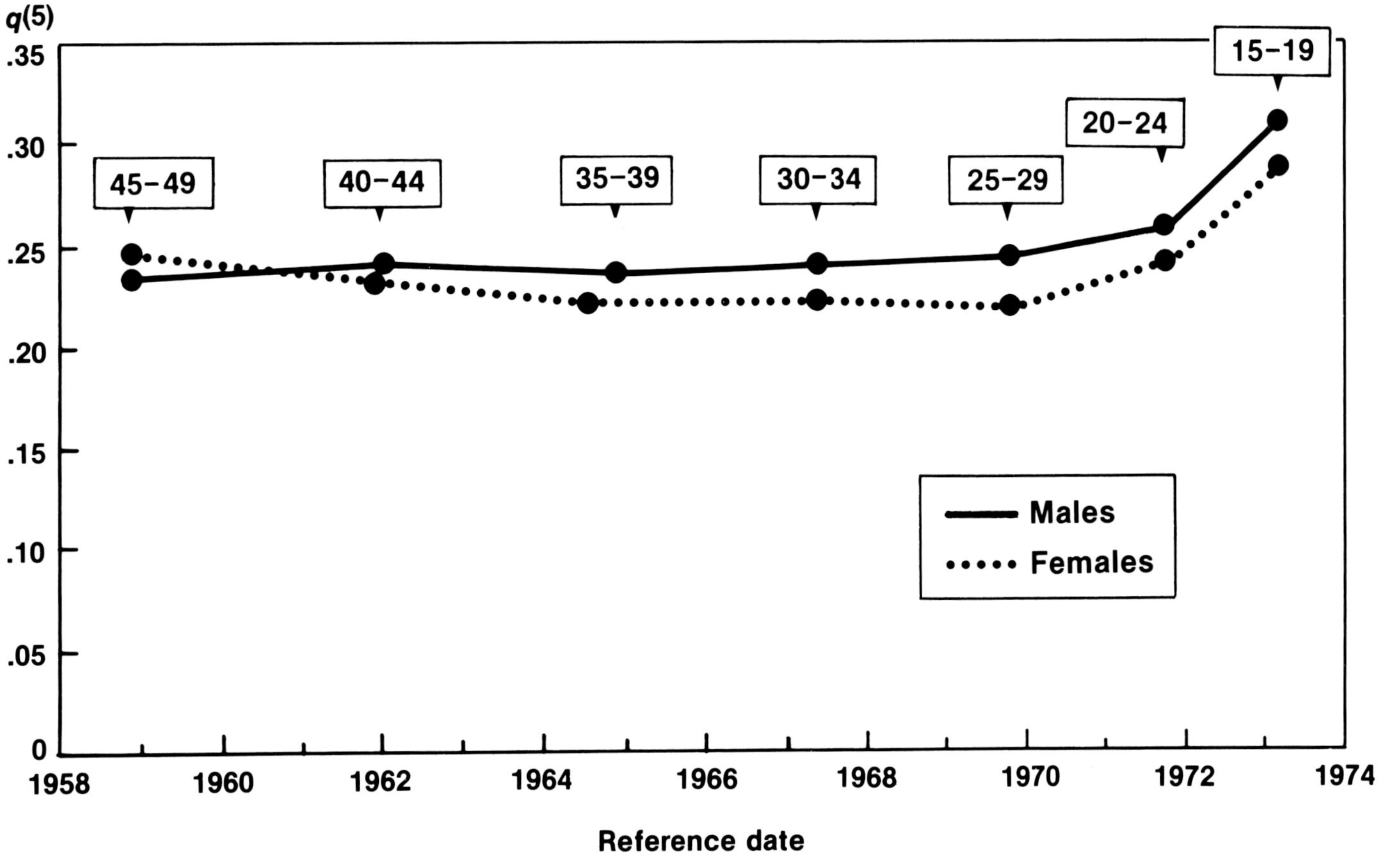

Sources: Tables 8 and 9.

As in the case of the data referring to both sexes, the estimates derived from information provided by younger women (age groups 15-19 and 20-24) seem to be biased upward and must be rejected. From the remaining estimates, it can be concluded that during the 1962-1970 period under-five mortality among males in Bangladesh remained mostly constant at a level of 238 or 239 deaths per 1,000 births, while that among females might have decreased slightly, from about 234 deaths per 1,000 births around 1962 to about 220 towards the end of the decade. The existence of such a decline may be further supported by the fact that our earlier analysis of sex ratios at birth showed that female children were under-reported among older women. If, as is likely, the omitted female children were dead children, the estimates for females derived from women aged 40-44 or 45-49 would underestimate mortality and hide or minimize the decline that has taken place. It is likely that the same biases may be operating on the estimates for males, especially if one accepts as improbable the reversal of the sex differential implied by the estimates derived from the reports of women aged 45-49.

If the conclusion that female mortality declined is accepted on the basis of the arguments presented above, the earlier conclusions regarding mortality levels for both sexes combined must be revised to reflect a decline in those levels, albeit slight, between the early and the late 1960s.

This example demonstrates the importance of analysing all available evidence before reaching definitive conclusions about the reliability of the different estimates yielded by the Brass method.

Chapter V

PALLONI-HELIGMAN VERSION OF THE BRASS METHOD

Another version of the Brass method was developed in the early 1980s by A. Palloni and L. Heligman (1986). It is based on the United Nations model life tables for developing countries and, like the Trussell version, produces estimates of the probabilities of dying from birth and of the time to which those probabilities refer. It differs from the Trussell version in that it uses information on births in a year in addition to the data required by the Brass method. The additional data are used to compute the mean age at maternity, an indicator of the average age difference between mothers and their children.

This chapter starts by describing the additional data requirements of the Palloni-Heligman version. It then describes the steps of the computational procedure to be followed in applying it and ends by providing a detailed example of its application to the case of Bangladesh.

DATA REQUIRED

The data required to apply the Palloni-Heligman version of the Brass method are essentially the same as those needed for the application of the Trussell version, namely:

1. Number of children ever born classified by age group of mother;

2. Number of children dead classified by age group of mother;

3. Total number of women (irrespective of marital or reporting status) classified by age.

However, the Palloni-Heligman version requires an additional set of information:

4. Number of births occurring in a given year classified by age group of mother

Information on births in a year is used to estimate an indicator of the timing of child-bearing, namely, the mean age at maternity (that is, the mean age of the mothers of the children born in a particular period), denoted by M. When information on births is not available, a rough estimate of M may be used in applying the Palloni-Heligman version (a convenient estimate is $M = 27$).

The first three items of data listed above can be compiled using the worksheets presented in displays 6 and 7 of chapter II. To compile the data on births in a given year, display 9 has been prepared. Note that the information on births need not be available by sex of child and that it is important to establish whether the information was derived from a registration system or from a survey or census. Generally, it is assumed that a registration system records births as they occur and consequently that

the age of mother recorded by the registration system is her age at the time of the birth. Surveys, on the other hand, usually obtain the necessary information on births by asking whether or not a woman gave birth during the year preceding interview. When such data are later tabulated by a woman's age at the time of interview, a systematic bias is introduced in the timing of births. To correct that bias, it is assumed that births occur uniformly throughout the year. Hence, on average, women aged 17, say, at the time of interview would have been aged 16.5 at the time they gave birth. For that reason the exact-age groups listed in the lower panel of display 9 referring to census or survey data have been shifted back half a year.

COMPUTATIONAL PROCEDURE

The application of the Palloni-Heligman version of the Brass method is very similar to that of the Trussell version. To maintain comparability with the latter in the numbering of steps, step 3 is divided here into two parts: 3 (*a*) and 3 (*b*).

Step 1. *Calculation of average parity per woman*

Average parity is the average number of children ever borne by women in a given five-year age group. It is calculated as

$$P(i) = \frac{CEB(i)}{FP(i)} \qquad (5.1)$$

where $P(i)$ is the average parity of women of age group i, $CEB(i)$ is the total number of children ever borne by these women, and $FP(i)$ is the total number of women in the age group irrespective of their marital or reporting status. Although parity values are needed only for age groups 15-19, 20-24 and 25-29—P(1), P(2) and P(3), respectively—it is worth calculating the whole set up to age group 45-49 in order to check the quality of the basic data. Note that the denominator, $FP(i)$, should include even those women who did not respond to the questions on children ever born (those of not-stated parity). Their inclusion is justified on the assumption that they are childless.

Step 2. *Calculation of the proportions dead among children ever born*

The proportion of children dead is given simply by the ratio of the total number of dead children to the total number of children ever born (including those who have died) for each age group of women. Thus,

$$D(i) = \frac{CD(i)}{CEB(i)} \qquad (5.2)$$

**Display 9. Worksheet for the compilation of data on births in a year by age group of mother
for the Palloni-Heligman version of the Brass method**

Source and reported age group of mother		Exact-age group of mother at birth of child[a]	Midpoint of exact-age group	Births in a year
Vital registration	15-19	[15,20)	17.5	
	20-24	[20,25)	22.5	
	25-29	[25,30)	27.5	
	30-34	[30,35)	32.5	
	35-39	[35,40)	37.5	
	40-44	[40,45)	42.5	
	45-49	[45,50)	47.5	
Census or survey	15-19	[14.5,19.5)	17	
	20-24	[19.5,24.5)	22	
	25-29	[24.5,29.5)	27	
	30-34	[29.5,34.5)	32	
	35-39	[34.5,39.5)	37	
	40-44	[39.5,44.5)	42	
	45-49	[44.5,49.5)	47	

[a]The notation [x,y) indicates that exact ages at the time women gave birth range from *x* to *y*, exclusive of the latter, that is, age *y* is not quite reached.

where $D(i)$ is the proportion of children dead for women of the age group i, $CD(i)$ is the number of dead children reported by those women and $CEB(i)$ is the number of children ever borne by those women.

Step 3. *Calculation of the mean age at maternity, M (Palloni-Heligman version only)*

The value of the mean age at maternity, M, is estimated from the number of births occurring in a given year classified by age group of mother. As indicated earlier, when those data are compiled for use in the estimation procedure, it is important to establish whether they were obtained from vital registration (a registration system) or from a census or survey.

M is calculated by multiplying the midpoint of each age group by the number of births to women in that age group, summing the resulting products, and then dividing the sum by the total number of births (excluding those to women of not-stated age). Thus,

$$M = \frac{\sum_{i=1}^{7} (B(i)\, mp(i))}{\sum_{i=1}^{7} B(i)}$$

where the symbol Σ denotes sum, $B(i)$ denotes the number of births to women in age group i and $mp(i)$ is the midpoint in years of age group i.

The values of $mp(i)$ are shown in display 9 and clearly depend on the type of exact-age group being dealt with. The term "exact-age group" is used here to denote the true range of variation of the ages of mother in each reported age group. Generally, women belonging to a given age group, say 20-24, are all those whose age at

35

last birthday was 20, 21, 22, 23 or 24, that is, women whose exact ages may vary anywhere from 20.0 to 24.99 . . . without quite reaching 25. The notation [20,25) is used to denote that range of exact ages. The midpoint of that range is 22.5 years.

As noted above, when the data on births in a year are obtained from a vital registration system, it can be assumed that the reported age of mother is her age at the time she gave birth. In contrast, in surveys or censuses gathering information on the births occurring during the year immediately preceding interview, mothers were on average half a year younger at the birth of their reported children than at the time of interview. Hence, as shown in display 9, the exact-age groups of mothers are shifted back by half a year—for example [19.5,24.5) rather than

[20,25). As indicated in that display, the midpoints of those intervals are also moved back by half a year.

Step 3 (b).   *Calculation of the multipliers, k(i)*

The basic estimation equation for the Palloni-Heligman version is the same as for the Trussell version shown in equation 4.3:

$$q(x) = k(i) D(i) \qquad (5.4)$$

but the equation to calculate $k(i)$ now includes M as input:

$$k(i) = a(i) + b(i) \frac{P(1)}{P(2)} + c(i) \frac{P(2)}{P(3)} + d(i) M \qquad (5.5)$$

Table 10 shows the coefficients $a(i)$, $b(i)$, $c(i)$ and $d(i)$ for the seven age groups of women, from ages 15-19

TABLE 10.   COEFFICIENTS FOR THE ESTIMATION OF CHILD-MORTALITY MULTIPLIERS, $k(i)$, PALLONI-HELIGMAN VERSION OF THE BRASS METHOD, USING THE UNITED NATIONS MORTALITY MODELS

Model	Age group of mother (1)	Age group Index i (2)	Age x of children (3)	Coefficients			
				a(i) (4)	b(i) (5)	c(i) (6)	d(i) (7)
Latin American	15-19	1	1	0.6892	−1.6937	0.6464	0.0106
	20-24	2	2	1.3625	−0.3778	−0.2892	−0.0041
	25-29	3	3	1.0877	0.0197	−0.2986	0.0024
	30-34	4	5	0.7500	0.0532	−0.1106	0.0115
	35-39	5	10	0.5605	0.0222	0.0170	0.0171
	40-44	6	15	0.5024	0.0028	0.0048	0.0180
	45-49	7	20	0.5326	0.0052	0.0256	0.0168
Chilean	15-19	1	1	0.8274	−1.5854	0.5949	0.0097
	20-24	2	2	1.3129	−0.2457	−0.2329	−0.0031
	25-29	3	3	1.0632	0.0196	−0.1996	0.0021
	30-34	4	5	0.8236	0.0293	−0.0684	0.0081
	35-39	5	10	0.6895	0.0068	0.0032	0.0119
	40-44	6	15	0.6098	−0.0014	0.0166	0.0141
	45-49	7	20	0.5615	0.0040	0.0073	0.0159
South Asian	15-19	1	1	0.6749	−1.7580	0.6805	0.0109
	20-24	2	2	1.3716	−0.3652	−0.2966	−0.0041
	25-29	3	3	1.0899	0.0299	−0.2887	0.0024
	30-34	4	5	0.7694	0.0548	−0.0934	0.0108
	35-39	5	10	0.6156	0.0231	0.0298	0.0149
	40-44	6	15	0.6077	0.0040	0.0573	0.0141
	45-49	7	20	0.6952	0.0018	0.0306	0.0109
Far Eastern	15-19	1	1	0.7194	−1.3143	0.5432	0.0093
	20-24	2	2	1.2671	−0.2996	−0.2105	−0.0029
	25-29	3	3	1.0668	0.0017	−0.2424	0.0019
	30-34	4	5	0.7833	0.0307	−0.1103	0.0098
	35-39	5	10	0.5765	0.0068	−0.0202	0.0165
	40-44	6	15	0.4115	0.0014	0.0083	0.0213
	45-49	7	20	0.3071	0.0111	0.0129	0.0251
General	15-19	1	1	0.7210	−1.4686	0.5746	0.0095
	20-24	2	2	1.3115	−0.3360	−0.2475	−0.0034
	25-29	3	3	1.0768	0.0109	−0.2695	0.0021
	30-34	4	5	0.7682	0.0439	−0.1090	0.0105
	35-39	5	10	0.5769	0.0176	0.0038	0.0165
	40-44	6	15	0.4845	0.0034	0.0036	0.0187
	45-49	7	20	0.4760	0.0071	0.0246	0.0189

Estimation equations:

$$k(i) = a(i) + b(i) \frac{P(1)}{P(2)} + c(i) \frac{P(2)}{P(3)} + d(i)M$$

$$q(x) = k(i)D(i)$$

Source: Alberto Palloni and Larry Heligman, "Re-estimation of structural parameters to obtain estimates of mortality in developing countries", *Population Bulletin of the United Nations*, No. 18 (United Nations publication, Sales No. E.85.XIII.6), table 2B, p. 17; figures in column 4 have been corrected.

through ages 45-49 $(i = 1, \ldots, 7)$, and for the five regional patterns of the United Nations models.

Step 4. *Calculation of the probabilities of dying by age x, q(x)*

Once $D(i)$ and $k(i)$ have been calculated for each age group i, estimates of $q(x)$ are obtained simply as their product, as already indicated in equation 5.4:

$$q(x) = k(i) D(i)$$

Step 5. *Calculation of the reference dates for q(x), t(i)*

An estimate of the time reference, $t(i)$, of each estimated $q(x)$ value is calculated by applying the coefficients in table 11 to the parity ratios $P(1)/P(2)$ and $P(2)/P(3)$ in the same way as for the Trussell version:

$$t(i) = e(i) + f(i) \frac{P(1)}{P(2)} + g(i) \frac{P(2)}{P(3)} \qquad (5.6)$$

However, in the Palloni-Heligman version, the values of $e(i)$, $f(i)$ and $g(i)$ appearing in equation 5.6 are based on the United Nations models (see table 11). Once the $t(i)$ values are calculated, they can be converted into reference dates by subtracting them from the reference date of the census or survey, as illustrated below.

Step 6. *Conversion to a common index*

Steps 4 and 5 provide estimates of $q(x)$ for ages x of 1, 2, 3, 5, 10, 15 and 20 and of $t(i)$, the number of years before the survey or census to which each estimate applies. In order to analyse trends and facilitate comparison both within and between data sets, each estimated $q(x)$ is converted to a single measure. Although any index from the model-life-table family can be used, it is suggested that a measure of child mortality that is not particularly sensitive to the pattern of mortality be

TABLE 11. COEFFICIENTS FOR THE ESTIMATION OF THE TIME REFERENCE, $t(i)$,[a] FOR VALUES OF $q(x)$, PALLONI-HELIGMAN VERSION OF THE BRASS METHOD, USING THE UNITED NATIONS MORTALITY MODELS

Model	Age group of mother (1)	Age group index i (2)	Estimated $q(x)$ (3)	Coefficients $e(i)$ (4)	$f(i)$ (5)	$g(i)$ (6)
Latin American	15-19	1	$q(1)$	1.1703	0.5129	−0.3850
	20-24	2	$q(2)$	1.6955	4.1320	−0.1635
	25-29	3	$q(3)$	1.8296	2.9020	3.4707
	30-34	4	$q(5)$	2.1783	−2.5688	9.0883
	35-39	5	$q(10)$	2.8836	−10.3282	15.4301
	40-44	6	$q(15)$	4.4580	−17.1809	20.4296
	45-49	7	$q(20)$	6.9351	−19.3871	23.4007
Chilean	15-19	1	$q(1)$	1.3092	1.9474	−0.7982
	20-24	2	$q(2)$	1.6897	4.6176	−0.0173
	25-29	3	$q(3)$	1.8368	2.6370	4.0305
	30-34	4	$q(5)$	2.2036	−3.3520	9.9233
	35-39	5	$q(10)$	2.9955	−11.4013	16.3441
	40-44	6	$q(15)$	4.7734	−17.8850	20.8883
	45-49	7	$q(20)$	7.4495	−19.0513	23.0529
South Asian	15-19	1	$q(1)$	1.1922	0.7940	−0.5425
	20-24	2	$q(2)$	1.7173	4.3117	−0.1653
	25-29	3	$q(3)$	1.8631	2.8767	3.5848
	30-34	4	$q(5)$	2.1808	−2.7219	9.3705
	35-39	5	$q(10)$	2.7654	−10.8808	16.2255
	40-44	6	$q(15)$	4.1378	−18.6219	22.2390
	45-49	7	$q(20)$	6.4885	−22.2001	26.4911
Far Eastern	15-19	1	$q(1)$	1.2779	1.5714	−0.6994
	20-24	2	$q(2)$	1.7471	4.2638	−0.0752
	25-29	3	$q(3)$	1.9107	2.7285	3.5881
	30-34	4	$q(5)$	2.3172	−2.6259	9.0238
	35-39	5	$q(10)$	3.2087	−9.8891	14.7339
	40-44	6	$q(15)$	5.1141	−15.3263	18.2507
	45-49	7	$q(20)$	7.6383	−15.5739	19.7669
General	15-19	1	$q(1)$	1.2136	0.9740	−0.5247
	20-24	2	$q(2)$	1.7025	4.1569	−0.1232
	25-29	3	$q(3)$	1.8360	2.8632	3.5220
	30-34	4	$q(5)$	2.1882	−2.6521	9.1961
	35-39	5	$q(10)$	2.9682	−10.3053	15.3161
	40-44	6	$q(15)$	4.6526	−16.6920	19.8534
	45-49	7	$q(20)$	7.1425	−18.3021	22.4168

Estimation equation:

$$t(i) = e(i) + f(i) \frac{P(1)}{P(2)} + g(i) \frac{P(2)}{P(3)}$$

Source: Alberto Palloni and Larry Heligman, "Re-estimation of structural parameters to obtain estimates of mortality in developing countries", *Population Bulletin of the United Nations*, No. 18 (United Nations publication, Sales No. E.85.XIII.6), table 5A, p. 19.

[a] Number of years prior to the survey.

selected. The common index recommended is under-five mortality, $q(5)$.

The $q(x)$ values corresponding to the model-life-table family being considered can be used to carry out the required conversions. The tables in annex II contain the necessary values of $q(x)$ ordered by mortality level and expectation of life for each of the United Nations models and for males, females and both sexes separately. The actual conversion is carried out by linear interpolation between tabulated values, as explained below.

Suppose that an estimated value of $q(x)$, denoted by $q^e(x)$, is to be converted to the corresponding $q^c(5)$ where $x \neq 5$. For a given model-life-table family and sex, it is first necessary to identify the mortality levels with $q(x)$ values that enclose the estimated value, $q^e(x)$. Thus, the task is to identify in the appropriate table of annex II levels j and $j + 1$ such that

$$q^j(x) > q^e(x) > q^{j+1}(x) \qquad (5.7)$$

where $q^j(x)$ and $q^{j+1}(x)$ are the model values of $q(x)$ for levels j and $j + 1$, respectively, and $q^e(x)$ is the estimated value. Then, the desired common index $q^c(5)$ is given by

$$q^c(5) = (1.0 - h) q^j(5) + h q^{j+1}(5) \qquad (5.8)$$

where h is the interpolation factor calculated in the following way:

$$h = \frac{q^e(x) - q^j(x)}{q^{j+1}(x) - q^j(x)} \qquad (5.9)$$

If the data on children ever born and children dead are for both sexes combined, the model $q^j(x)$ values should be taken from the tables for both sexes combined in annex II. If, however, the data are for male and female children separately, the estimated values of $q(x)$ will be sex-specific, and the conversion to a common index should use the model $q^j(x)$ values from the tables for the relevant sex also presented in annex II.

Step 7. *Interpolation and analysis of results*

Once seven estimates (one for each age group i of women) of the selected common index—$q^c(5)$—have been obtained, it is recommended that they be plotted against time. As noted in step 5, the $t(i)$ values can be converted into reference dates by subtracting them from the survey or census reference date (or the approximate midpoint of the field-work), and the $q^c(5)$ estimates can then be plotted against the resulting dates. Graphical presentation of the results is essential to assess the consistency and general trend of the estimates, as the example below illustrates.

A DETAILED EXAMPLE

Compilation of the data required

The 1974 Bangladesh Retrospective Survey of Fertility and Mortality will be used once more to provide an example. The data on children ever born and children dead and the total number of women have already been compiled in displays 6 and 7 (reproduced again here). In this example, estimates of the risks of dying in childhood will be estimated for male children. Hence, the data of interest are those referring to male children ever born and male children dead in display 6.

To apply the Palloni-Heligman version, it is also necessary to compile information on births occurring during a given year. Display 10 shows the published tabulation on that topic. Note that the 1974 Bangladesh survey gathered information on the time of occurrence of the most recent live birth of each ever-married woman and that such information was tabulated by year of occurrence. The analyst is thus apparently faced with a choice of which time period to use. Note that a woman who had a child in April 1972 and another one in March 1974 would report only the latter birth. Consequently the data for the period April 1972 to March 1973 do not cover all the births during that year. It is therefore necessary to use the most recent period—in this case April 1973 to March 1974, the year immediately preceding the survey. Because of the type of information gathered (the date of the most recent birth), only the most recent time period will cover all possible events (births) in a year.

The worksheet presented in display 9 may be used to compile the data on births in the year preceding the survey. Display 11 illustrates a completed worksheet. Note that data on births in a year for both sexes combined are adequate for the application of the method even when estimates of mortality by sex are desired.

Computational procedure

Step 1. *Calculation of average parity per woman*

Average parities are computed by dividing the number of children ever born by the total number of women, age group by age group. In this case, only male children ever born will be used, since male mortality is being estimated. As an example, the average parity of women aged 35-39, $P_m(5)$, where the subindex m indicates that only data on male children are used, is calculated below:

$$P_m(5) = \frac{5,435,726}{1,771,680} = 3.0681$$

The full set of parities in respect of male children is shown in column 3 of table 12. At the foot of the table, the values of the relevant parity ratios, $P_m(1)/P_m(2)$ and $P_m(2)/P_m(3)$ also are displayed. Note that, as in the case of both sexes combined, the average parity decreases from age group 40-44 to age group 45-49, which suggests the existence of omission errors.

Step 2. *Calculation of the proportions dead among children ever born*

As in the Trussell version, the proportions of children dead are calculated by dividing the number of children dead by the number of those ever born, for each age group of women. Again in this example, only male children are considered, and hence the subindex m is used. Thus, $D_m(5)$, the proportion of male children dead among those ever borne by women aged 35-39 is calculated as follows:

**Display 6. Second step in the compilation of data on children ever born
and children dead for Bangladesh**

Age group of mother	Children ever born (1) = (2) + (3) = (2) + (4) + (5)	Children dead (2) = (1) − (3) = (1) − (4) − (5)	Children surviving (3) = (4) + (5)	Children living at home (4)	Children living elsewhere (5)
Both sexes					
15-19	1 160 919	215 365		921 227	24 327
20-24	4 901 382	997 384		3 820 649	83 349
25-29	9 085 852	1 937 955		6 927 908	219 989
30-34	9 910 256	2 261 196		7 126 473	522 587
35-39	10 384 001	2 490 168		6 974 267	919 566
40-44	9 164 329	2 415 023		5 472 460	1 276 846
45-49	6 905 673	1 959 544		3 664 328	1 281 801
Male					
15-19	597 248	117 165		469 036	11 047
20-24	2 507 018	529 877		1 938 220	38 921
25-29	4 675 978	1 047 294		3 545 904	82 780
30-34	5 109 487	1 204 582		3 780 859	124 046
35-39	5 435 726	1 333 957		3 925 071	176 698
40-44	4 883 599	1 291 745		3 323 724	268 130
45-49	3 714 957	1 030 737		2 393 149	291 071
Female					
15-19	563 671	98 200		452 191	13 280
20-24	2 394 364	467 507		1 882 429	44 428
25-29	4 409 874	890 661		3 382 004	137 209
30-34	4 800 769	1 056 614		3 345 614	398 541
35-39	4 948 275	1 156 211		3 049 196	742 868
40-44	4 280 780	1 123 278		2 148 736	1 008 716
45-49	3 190 716	928 807		1 271 179	990 730

Source: Bangladesh, Census Commission, *Report on the 1974 Bangladesh Retrospective Survey of Fertility and Mortality* (Dacca, 1977), table 8, p. 37 (reproduced in display 3 above).

39

Display 7. Compilation of data on the total number of women by age group
for Bangladesh

Age group of women	Total number of women (1) = (2) + (3) = (4) + (5)	Ever-married women (2)	Single women (3)	Women of stated parity (4)	Women of not-stated parity (5)
15-19	3 014 706				
20-24	2 653 155				
25-29	2 607 009				
30-34	2 015 663				
35-39	1 771 680				
40-44	1 479 575				
45-49	1 135 129				

Source: Bangladesh, Census Commission, *Report on the 1974 Bangladesh Retrospective Survey of Fertility and Mortality* (Dacca, 1977), table 3, p. 28 (reproduced in display 4 above).

$$D_m(5) = \frac{1,333,957}{5,435,726} = .2454$$

The complete set of proportions dead is displayed in column 4 of table 12. Note that, as expected, the proportion dead increases with age of mother.

Step 3 (a). *Calculation of the mean age at maternity, M (Palloni-Heligman version only)*

The mean age at maternity is calculated using the data compiled in display 11. As equation 5.3 states, M is the ratio of two quantities: the sum of the products of births times the midpoints of the age groups of mothers, and the sum of births. Both are calculated below:

$$\sum_{i=1}^{7} B(i)\, mp(i) = (320,406)(17) + (609,271)(22)$$
$$+ (561,493)(27) + (367,833)(32)$$
$$+ (237,297)(37) + (95,356)(42)$$
$$+ (38,124)(47) = 60,358,600$$

$$\sum_{i=1}^{7} B(i) = 320,406 + 609,271 + 561,493$$
$$+ 367,833 + 237,297 + 95,356$$
$$+ 38,124 = 2,229,780$$

Then

$$M = \frac{60,358,600}{2,229,780} = 27.07$$

Step 3 (b). *Calculation of the multipliers, k(i)*

Table 10 shows the values of the regression coefficients $a(i)$, $b(i)$, $c(i)$ and $d(i)$ needed to calculate the multipliers $k(i)$ for each regional pattern of the United Nations model life tables. In this example, the South Asian pattern will be used. As equation 5.5 shows, for each age group i, $k(i)$ is computed as the sum of $a(i)$, the product of $b(i)$ and $P(1)/P(2)$, that of $c(i)$ and $P(2)/P(3)$, and that of $d(i)$ and M. Thus, for age group 5, in which women are aged 35-39,

$$k(5) = .6156 + (.0231)(.2097)$$
$$+ (.0298)(.5268) + (.0149)(27.07)$$
$$= 1.0395$$

Values of $k(i)$ for all age groups are shown in column 5 of table 12. Note that, as in the Trussell version, all values of $k(i)$ are close to 1.0.

Step 4. *Calculation of the probabilities of dying by age x, q(x)*

The probabilities of dying by exact age x are computed by multiplying the proportions dead $D_m(i)$ by the corresponding multipliers $k(i)$. To estimate $q_m(10)$, for example,

$$q_m(10) = (1.0395)(0.2454) = .255$$

The full set of $q_m(x)$ estimates is shown in column 7 of table 12.

Display 10.   Tabulation of data on births in a year as appearing in the report on the
1974 Bangladesh Retrospective Survey of Fertility and Mortality

BANGLADESH CENSUS 1974 RETROSPECTIVE SURVEY OF FERTILITY AND MORTALITY

BANGLADESH   DE FACTO

TABLE 10.   EVER-MARRIED WOMEN BY AGE GROUP, DATE OF LAST BIRTH AND SURVIVAL OF CHILD

	AGE GROUP	TOTAL WOMEN	CHILDLESS WOMEN	APRIL 73–MARCH 74	APRIL 72–MARCH 73	BEFORE APRIL 72	1973 N.M.	1972 N.M.	NOT STATED
TOTAL	UNDER 15	315 530	271 224	6 842	3 896	16 563	408	757	15 840
	15–19	2 031 604	1 166 887	320 406	219 069	261 832	19 769	16 649	26 992
	20–24	2 530 026	431 225	609 271	492 384	878 863	33 199	37 224	47 860
	25–29	2 577 574	159 934	561 493	503 986	1 222 507	36 967	47 792	44 895
	30–34	2 005 083	79 049	367 833	326 551	1 131 739	27 994	31 909	40 008
	35–39	1 767 440	51 649	237 297	223 428	1 181 078	10 852	18 633	44 503
	40–44	1 475 299	49 573	95 356	105 376	1 157 209	6 681	11 657	49 447
	45–49	1 130 992	39 453	38 124	36 784	948 263	2 970	4 179	61 219
	50–54	1 043 611	40 848	8 702	14 775	897 732	1 233	4 147	76 174
	55+	2 249 264	103 726	6 599	6 775	1 845 939	1 139	2 049	283 037
	N.S.	819	204			615			
	TOTAL	17 127 242	2 393 772	2 251 923	1 933 024	9 542 340	141 212	174 996	689 975
CHILD ALIVE	UNDER 15	24 863		5 635	3 097	13 197	408	757	1 769
	15–19	759 221		280 716	200 411	236 600	17 643	15 637	8 214
	20–24	1 905 774		552 453	464 519	808 529	29 227	35 840	15 206
	25–29	2 214 326		513 568	473 360	1 133 773	35 018	46 600	12 007
	30–34	1 745 901		334 935	306 445	1 036 413	27 039	30 876	10 193
	35–39	1 534 253		213 951	207 410	1 075 709	10 038	18 050	9 095
	40–44	1 236 604		86 464	96 434	1 024 122	6 489	10 042	13 053
	45–49	907 485		33 241	32 270	816 039	2 970	3 561	19 404
	50–54	807 333		7 738	13 373	750 376	1 233	3 943	30 670
	55+	1 528 577		4 887	5 219	1 410 130	935	1 635	105 771
	N.S.	204				204			
	TOTAL	12 664 541		2 033 588	1 802 538	8 305 092	131 000	166 941	225 382
CHILD DEAD	UNDER 15	6 588		1 207	799	3 366			1 216
	15–19	99 582		39 690	18 658	24 821	2 126	1 012	13 275
	20–24	188 309		56 818	27 865	70 334	3 972	1 384	27 936
	25–29	200 173		47 925	30 626	88 551	1 949	1 192	29 930
	30–34	177 766		32 898	20 106	95 119	955	1 033	27 655
	35–39	179 187		23 346	16 018	105 369	814	583	33 057
	40–44	186 209		8 892	8 942	132 691	192	1 615	33 877
	45–49	181 285		4 883	4,514	131 848		618	39 422
	50–54	192 337		964	1 402	147 164		204	42 603
	55+	598 805		1 712	1 556	435 422	204	414	159 497
	N.S.	411				411			
	TOTAL	2 010 652		218 335	130 486	1 235 096	10 212	8 055	408 468
CHILD N.S.	UNDER 15	12 855							12 855
	15–19	5 914				411			5 503
	20–24	4 718							4 718
	25–29	3 141				183			2 958
	30–34	2 367				207			2 160
	35–39	2 351							2 351
	40–44	2 913				396			2 517
	45–49	2 769				376			2 393
	50–54	3 093				192			2 901
	55+	18 156				387			17 769
	N.S.								
	TOTAL	58 277				2 152			56 125

Source: Bangladesh, Census Commission, *Report on the 1974 Bangladesh Retrospective Survey of Fertility and Mortality* (Dacca, 1977), p. 39.

TABLE 12.   APPLICATION OF THE PALLONI-HELIGMAN VERSION OF THE BRASS METHOD TO DATA ON MALES
FROM THE 1974 BANGLADESH RETROSPECTIVE SURVEY

Age group of mother (1)	Age group index (i) (2)	Average parity $P_m(i)$ (3)	Proportion dead $D_m(i)$ (4)	Multiplier $k(i)$ (5)	Age x (6)	Probability of dying by age x, $q_m(x)$ (7)	Time reference $t(i)$ (8)	Reference date (9)	Common index $q_m^c(5)$ (10)
15–19	1	0.1981	.1962	0.9598	1	.188	1.1	1973.2	.311
20–24	2	0.9449	.2114	1.0278	2	.217	2.5	1971.8	.268
25–29	3	1.7936	.2240	1.0091	3	.226	4.4	1969.9	.249
30–34	4	2.5349	.2358	1.0240	5	.241	6.5	1967.8	.241
35–39	5	3.0681	.2454	1.0395	10	.255	9.0	1965.3	.237
40–44	6	3.3007	.2645	1.0204	15	.270	11.9	1962.4	.244
45–49	7	3.2727	.2775	1.0069	20	.279	15.8	1958.5	.245

$P_m(1)/P_m(2) = .2097$
$P_m(2)/P_m(3) = .5268$

$M = 27.07$ years
Multipliers based on South Asian model.

41

**Display 11. Compilation of data on births in a year by age group of mother
for Bangladesh**

	Source and reported age group of mother	Exact-age group of mother at birth of child[a]	Midpoint of exact-age group	Births in a year
Vital registration	15-19	[15,20)	17.5	
	20-24	[20,25)	22.5	
	25-29	[25,30)	27.5	
	30-34	[30,35)	32.5	
	35-39	[35,40)	37.5	
	40-44	[40,45)	42.5	
	45-49	[45,50)	47.5	
Census or survey	15-19	[14.5,19.5)	17	320 406
	20-24	[19.5,24.5)	22	609 271
	25-29	[24.5,29.5)	27	561 493
	30-34	[29.5,34.5)	32	367 833
	35-39	[34.5,39.5)	37	237 297
	40-44	[39.5,44.5)	42	95 356
	45-49	[44.5,49.5)	47	38 124

Source: Bangladesh, Census Commission, *Report on the 1974 Bangladesh Retrospective Survey of Fertility and Mortality* (Dacca, 1977), table 10, p. 29 (reproduced in display 10 above).

[a] The notation [*x,y*) indicates that exact ages at the time women gave birth range from *x* to *y*, exclusive of the latter, that is, age *y* is not quite reached.

Step 5. *Calculation of the reference dates for* q(x), t(i)

Again using the South Asian model, the coefficients needed for the estimation of $t(i)$ are obtained from the third panel of table 11. Following equation 5.6, $t(5)$ is calculated below:

$$t(5) = 2.7654 + (-10.8808)(.2097)$$

$$+ (16.2255)(.5268) = 9.01$$

That is, the estimated value of $q_m(10)$ refers to a period approximately 9 years before the survey. A more illuminating reference date is obtained by subtracting each $t(i)$ value from the survey's reference date expressed in decimal form—1974.3 in this case (see step 5 of the detailed example for the Trussell version). Hence, the reference date for $q_m(10)$ is:

$$1974.3 - 9.0 = 1965.3$$

All estimated values of $t(i)$ and the reference dates derived from them are presented, respectively, in columns 8 and 9 of table 12.

Step 6. *Conversion to a common index*

The estimates of $q_m(x)$ for different values of x are now converted into equivalent estimates of $q_m^c(5)$ using the South Asian family of United Nations model life tables for males. Consider, for example, the estimated probability of dying by age 10, $q_m^e(10) = .225$. Using table A.II.3, one can identify the two life-table levels having $q(10)$ values such that:

$$q_m^j(10) > q_m^e(10) > q_m^{j+1}(10)$$

Those values are $q_m^{14}(10)$, which equals .25794 and whose $q_m^{14}(5)$ equivalent is .23986, and $q_m^{15}(10)$, which equals .24715 and has a corresponding $q_m^{15}(5)$ of .22989. Using equation 5.9, the interpolation factor h is obtained as follows:

$$h = \frac{.25500 - .25794}{.24715 - .25794} = .2725$$

Then, making use of equation 5.8, the desired $q^c(5)$ is calculated in the following way:

42

$$q_m^c(5) = (1.0 - (.2725)(.23986) + (.2725)(.22989)$$
$$= .237$$

The full set of $q_m^c(5)$ equivalents is shown in column 10 of table 12.

Step 7. *Interpretation and analysis of results*

The estimated probabilities of surviving by age 5, $q_m^c(5)$, are plotted against their respective reference dates in figure 9. Note that the general trend of the resulting curve is very similar to that obtained using the Trussell version with model South (see table 8 and figure 8). Once more, under-five mortality, $q(5)$, varies within a fairly narrow range between 1958 and 1970, only to rise sharply for the most recent period (1970-1973). Again, this apparent increase is probably spurious, since it is likely to be caused by the higher-than-average mortality characterizing the children of younger women.

On the other hand, estimates for the earliest period may be biased downward, since they are derived from information provided by older women. But the estimates for males considered in isolation do not provide clear evidence of the existence of such biases. If no further information were available, it would be relatively safe to conclude that male mortality changed little during the 1960s and to adopt as a reasonable estimate of its level the mean of the under-five mortality estimates associated with age groups 25-29, 30-34 and even 35-39, namely a $q_m(5)$ equal to .242 for the period 1965-1970. It should be noted that such a value is very close to that estimated in chapter IV using the Trussell version—a $q_m(5)$ of approximately .238 or .239 (see pp. 32-33). The following section will show that the sex differentials in mortality estimated using the United Nations South Asian model lead to the same conclusions reached when analysing the sex-specific estimates produced by the Coale-Demeny South model.

Figure 9. **Under-five mortality, $q(5)$, for males in Bangladesh, estimated using the South Asian model and the Palloni-Heligman version of the Brass method**

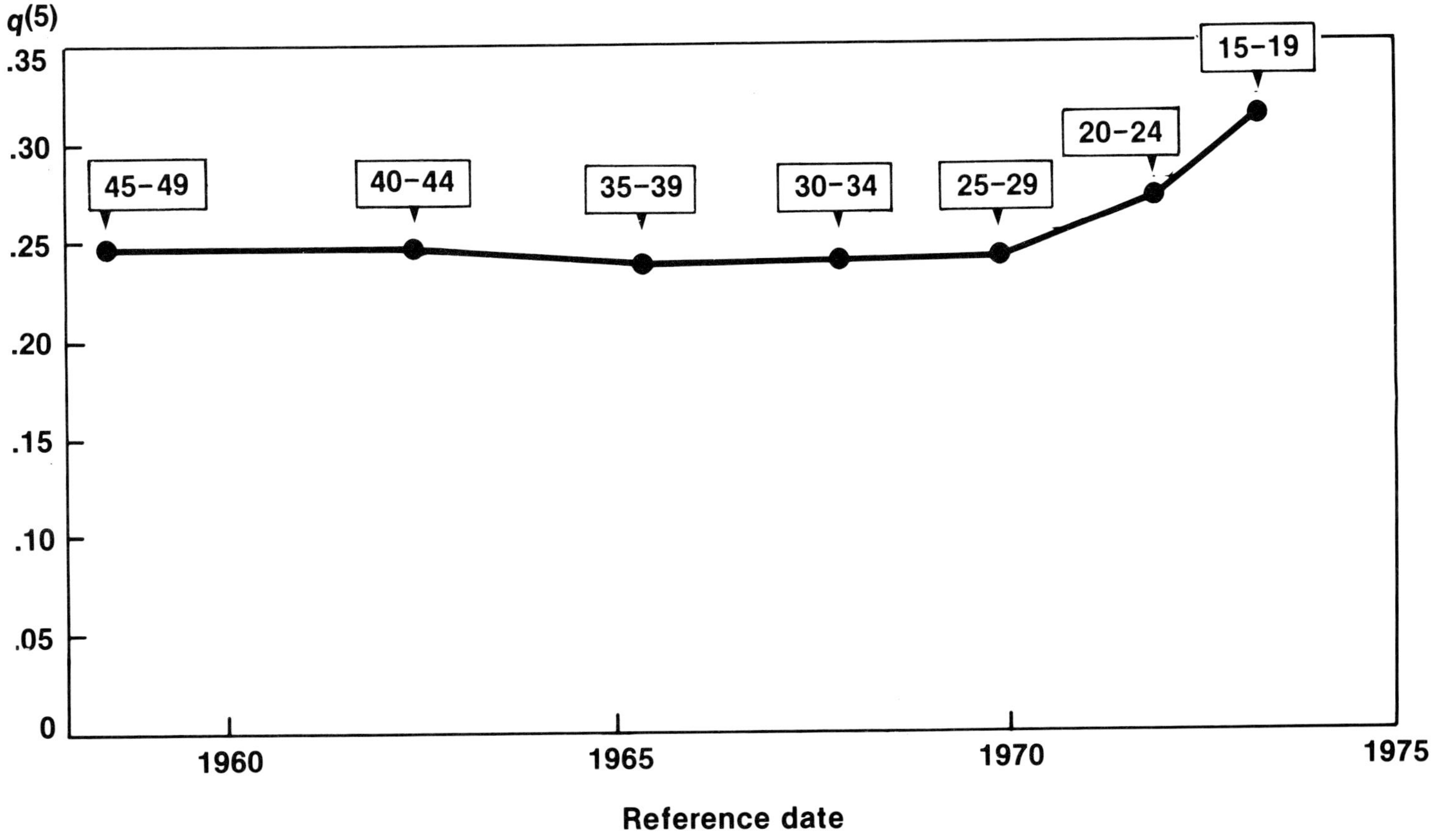

Source: Table 12.

TABLE 13. APPLICATION OF THE PALLONI-HELIGMAN VERSION OF THE BRASS METHOD TO DATA ON FEMALES FROM THE 1974 BANGLADESH RETROSPECTIVE SURVEY

Age group of mother (1)	Age group index (i) (2)	Average parity $P_f(i)$ (3)	Proportion dead $D_f(i)$ (4)	Multiplier $k(i)$ (5)	Age x (6)	Probability of dying by age x, $q_f(x)$ (7)	Time reference $t(i)$ (8)	Reference date (9)	Common index $q_f'(5)$ (10)
15-19......................	1	0.1897	.1742	0.9688	1	.169	1.1	1973.2	.296
20-24......................	2	0.9025	.1953	1.0267	2	.201	2.5	1971.8	.253
25-29......................	3	1.6916	.2020	1.0070	3	.203	4.4	1969.9	.226
30-34......................	4	2.3817	.2201	1.0233	5	.225	6.6	1967.7	.225
35-39......................	5	2.7930	.2337	1.0396	10	.243	9.2	1965.1	.225
40-44......................	6	2.8932	.2624	1.0208	15	.268	12.1	1962.2	.240
45-49......................	7	2.8109	.2911	1.0070	20	.293	16.0	1958.3	.251

$P_f(1)/P_f(2) = .2072$
$P_f(2)/P_f(3) = .5335$

$M = 27.07$ years
Multipliers based on South Asian model

Figure 10. Under-five mortality, $q(5)$, for males and females in Bangladesh, estimated using the South Asian model and the Palloni-Heligman version of the Brass method

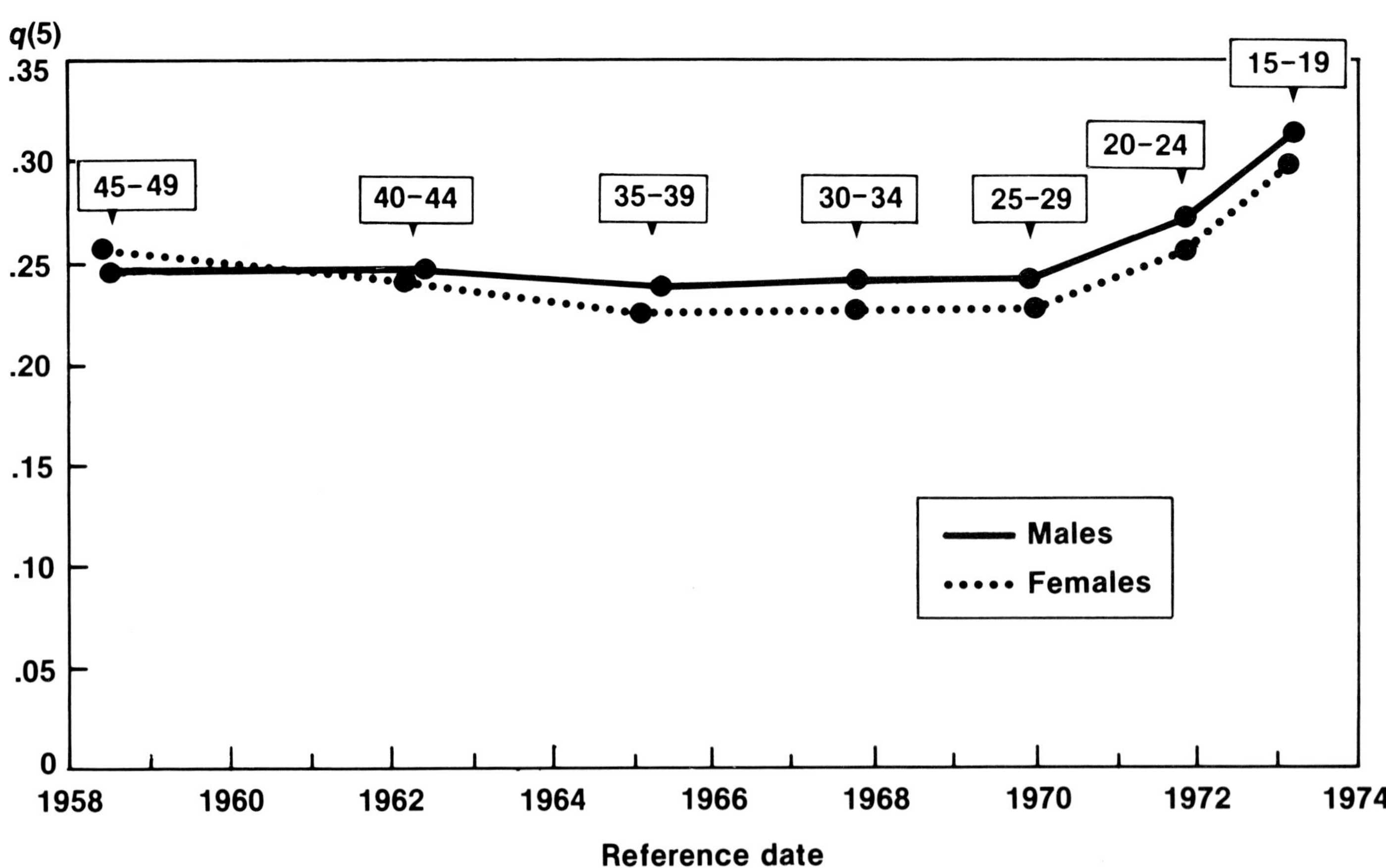

Sources: Tables 12 and 13.

Tables 13 and 14 present the estimates of $q(5)$ obtained by applying the Palloni-Heligman version of the Brass method to the Bangladesh data referring to females and to both sexes combined (using in all cases the South Asian model). In addition, figure 10 presents a graphical comparison of estimated under-five mortality by sex. Figure 10 should be compared with figure 8, which shows the estimates by sex yielded by the Trussell version. Both sets of estimates have the same overall characteristics: with the exception of estimates derived from the reports of women aged 45-49, the estimated under-five mortality of males is, as is generally the case in most countries of the world, higher than that of females. The reversal in the trend observed for age group 45-49 is likely to be caused by errors in the basic data and should be disregarded.

In both sets, the estimates for females show a somewhat clearer declining trend during the 1958-1970 period than those for males. According to the Palloni-Heligman estimates, under-five mortality among females may have declined from approximately .240 in 1962 to around .225-.226 in 1970. According to the Trussell version, the decline during the same period would have been from .234 to .218. The magnitude of both declines is nearly the same, though the starting and ending points differ slightly. Such consistency is determined both by the basic data and by the similarity of the South and South Asian patterns used to derive the estimates considered here. In the next chapter, the effects of choosing different mortality models in estimating mortality in childhood will be considered in some detail.

TABLE 14.   APPLICATION OF THE PALLONI-HELIGMAN VERSION OF THE BRASS METHOD TO DATA ON BOTH SEXES
FROM THE 1974 BANGLADESH RETROSPECTIVE SURVEY

Age group of mother (1)	Age group index (i) (2)	Average parity P(i) (3)	Proportion dead D(i) (4)	Multiplier k(i) (5)	Age x (6)	Probability of dying by age x, q(x) (7)	Time reference t(i) (8)	Reference date (9)	Common index q'(5) (10)
15-19	1	0.3851	.1855	0.9642	1	.179	1.1	1973.2	.304
20-24	2	1.8474	.2035	1.0272	2	.209	2.5	1971.8	.261
25-29	3	3.4852	.2133	1.0081	3	.215	4.4	1969.9	.238
30-34	4	4.9166	.2282	1.0273	5	.234	6.6	1967.7	.234
35-39	5	5.8611	.2398	1.0396	10	.249	9.1	1965.2	.231
40-44	6	6.1940	.2635	1.0206	15	.269	12.0	1962.3	.242
45-49	7	6.0836	.2838	1.0069	20	.286	15.9	1958.4	.248

$P(1)/P(2) = .2085$
$P(2)/P(3) = .5301$
$M = 27.07\,years$

Multipliers based on South Asian model
Sex ratio at birth $= 1.05$

Chapter VI

INTERPRETATION AND USE OF THE ESTIMATES YIELDED BY THE BRASS METHOD

Through selected examples, this chapter discusses some of the most common problems encountered in using the estimates yielded by the Brass method and offers guidance regarding possible solutions to them. The reader must be forewarned, however, about the tentative nature of the solutions proposed, since they respond to problems arising from the lack of reliable information on the incidence of mortality over time. In other words, the strategies described attempt to reduce remaining gaps in knowledge but cannot eliminate them altogether.

WHICH VERSION OF THE BRASS METHOD SHOULD ONE USE?

The reader who has become familiar with the Trussell and the Palloni-Heligman versions of the Brass method presented in chapters IV and V above is probably asking which version to use. To answer that question, it is necessary to determine the best model to use for a given population.

Consider again figures 5 and 6 in chapter I. Those figures illustrate how the mortality patterns in childhood of different populations vary and how the patterns of certain populations are close to a given mortality model and not to others. Thus, if one knew, for example, that the mortality pattern in childhood of a given country was close to the Chilean pattern, the answer to the question posed above would be immediate: use the Palloni-Heligman version of the estimation method with the Chilean model. Unfortunately, for most populations whose mortality in childhood needs to be estimated indirectly, it is not easy to establish the model that most closely approximates the prevailing pattern.

Demographers faced with this quandary have developed certain rationalizations to justify the use of different mortality models and, hence, of different methods. For instance, it has been argued that in populations practising prolonged breast-feeding, mortality in infancy—below age 1—is likely to be relatively low with respect to mortality at older childhood ages—from 1 to 5—and, consequently, that it would be appropriate to use model North (that is, the Trussell version). It has also been suggested that, in the absence of reliable information on the pattern of mortality in childhood, the use of "average" models such as West (Trussell version) or the General pattern (Palloni-Heligman version) would be adequate.

In practice, determining the best model to use for a given population is still more an art than a science, and it is common to find that different analysts use different models in estimating mortality in childhood for the same population.

Given this state of affairs, it is nevertheless important to provide the reader, first, with tools to test the adequacy of the different models when information on the pattern of mortality in childhood is available and, secondly, with some sense of the magnitude of the errors that may arise if the best model is not used during the estimation process. These points will be considered in the next two sections.

Use of information on the pattern of mortality in childhood to test the adequacy of mortality models

Available information on the pattern of mortality in childhood may take different forms, but only two possible variants will be considered here: (1) reasonably reliable estimates of infant and under-five mortality and (2) infant- and child-mortality estimates.

First, note that the two combinations mentioned above are equivalent, since under-five mortality, $q(5)$, may be derived from infant mortality, $q(1)$, and child mortality, ${}_4q_1$, as follows:

$$q(5) = q(1) + (1.0 - q(1)){}_4q_1 \qquad (6.1)$$

For example, in the case of Bangladesh, estimates of infant and child mortality may be obtained from the 1975-1976 survey carried out as part of the World Fertility Survey programme. The estimates referring to the 0-9 years preceding the survey and derived from the information gathered in the fertility histories of interviewed women are $q(1) = .13275$ and ${}_4q_1 = .09130$. Under-five mortality is then obtained as

$$q(5) = .13275 + (1.0 - .13275)(.09130) = .21193$$

The adequacy of available mortality models for representing mortality in Bangladesh can now be assessed algebraically, as well as graphically (see figures 5 and 6 in chapter I and annexes III and IV). The algebraic approach makes use of the tables in annexes I and II. It consists of using equations 5.7, 5.8 and 5.9 to find the $q(5)$ values associated with the estimated $q^e(1) = .13275$ for each of the mortality models available. For instance, according to model North for both sexes combined (see table A.I.9), the two values of $q(1)$ surrounding $q^e(1)$ are $q^{11}(1) = .14076$ and $q^{12}(1) = .12744$, whose corresponding values of under-five mortality are

$q^{11}(5) = .23793$ and $q^{12}(5) = .21533$. Hence, using equation 5.9,

$$h = \frac{.13275 - .14076}{.12744 - .14076} = .60135$$

and, using equation 5.8,

$$q^{N}(5) = (1.0 - .60135)(.23793) + (.60135)(.21533)$$
$$= .22434$$

Values of under-five mortality corresponding to the estimated $q^{e}(1)$ for all the available mortality models are presented in table 15, together with the ratios of those values to the estimated $q^{e}(5) = .21193$. Those ratios indicate how well the models fit the estimated values. A ratio of 1.0 indicates a perfect fit. In this case, both the South and the South Asian models provide an excellent fit, a conclusion already reached through the graphical comparison presented in chapter I.

Figure 11 presents a comparison of the estimates of mortality in childhood obtained in chapters IV and V by

TABLE 15. COMPARISON OF ESTIMATED INFANT AND UNDER-FIVE MORTALITY IN BANGLADESH[a] WITH THE AVAILABLE MORTALITY MODELS

Model	Model q(5) associated with $q^{e}(1) = .13275$	Ratio of model q(5) to $q^{e}(5)$[b]
Coale-Demeny models		
North	.22434	1.059
South	.21315	1.006
East	.17619	0.831
West	.20009	0.944
United Nations models		
Latin American	.22109	1.043
Chilean	.16863	0.796
South Asian	.21304	1.005
Far Eastern	.20727	0.978
General	.20922	0.987

[a]Estimates of $q^{e}(1)$ and $q^{e}(5)$ were obtained from the 1975-1976 World Fertility Survey.
[b]A ratio of 1.0 indicates a perfect fit between the country estimates and the mortality model.

Figure 11. Comparison of the estimates of under-five mortality in Bangladesh, obtained using models South and South Asian

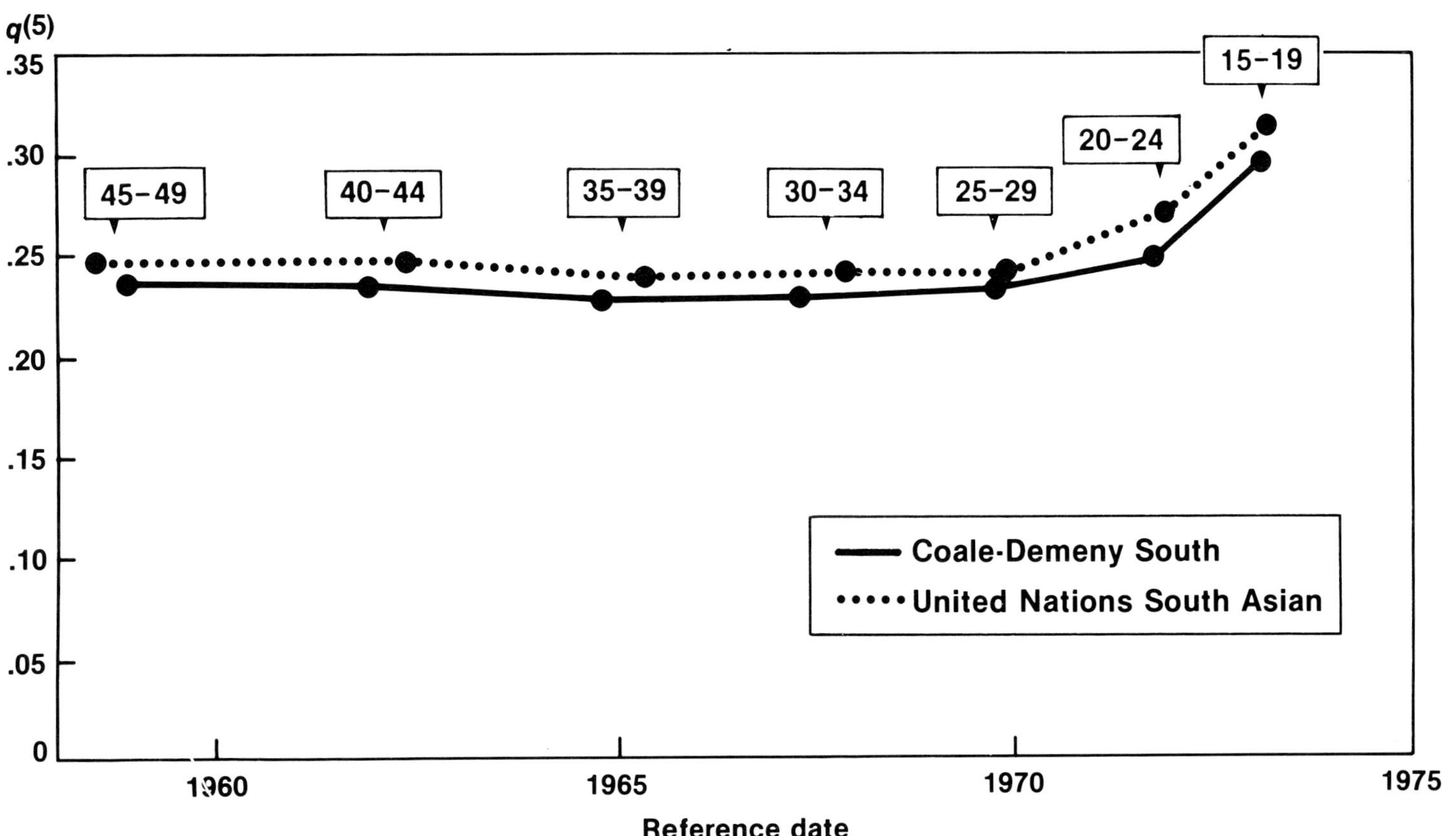

Sources: Tables 7 and 14.

using models South and South Asian in applying the Brass method. Note that, as expected, the estimates are very similar: they display a similar trend and are usually within 0.01 points of one another. This example shows that, if the appropriate model is used, it makes little difference whether estimates are derived using the Trussell or the Palloni-Heligman version of the Brass method.

What are the consequences of using the "wrong" model?

To assess the consequences of using the "wrong" model, let us suppose that the nine mortality models used in this *Guide* represent all possible mortality patterns in childhood. Although, strictly speaking, that assumption is false, since there are patterns of mortality in childhood that do not fit existing models (see chapter I), it nevertheless allows us to explore the sensitivity of different estimates to the choice of model.

To explore the variability of estimates with respect to the use of different models, we consider again the case of Bangladesh. Tables 16 and 17 present the complete set of infant and under-five mortality estimates for that country derived by applying the Trussell and Palloni-Heligman versions of the Brass method to the 1974 data classified by sex. Application of the estimation procedures discussed in this *Guide* potentially yields a total of 63 (or 7 × 9) estimates of under-five mortality. If data for males, females and both sexes combined are available, the number of estimates of under-five mortality is multiplied by 3, yielding 189 values. If, as in tables 16 and 17, more than one common index is used for exploratory or evaluation purposes, the number of estimates increases again, in this case doubling, to 378. It is useful for the reader to become familiar with the many possible estimates, since, with the widespread use of computers, arrays of the type presented in tables 16 and 17 are common. In fact, in the case at hand, those tables display only a subset of the estimates routinely produced by the QFIVE program.

Generally, graphical displays offer the best tool to analyse the various estimates available. Figures 12 and 13 display graphically the sets of estimates for both sexes combined produced by the Trussell and Palloni-Heligman versions, respectively. It is apparent from those figures that the estimates of under-five mortality, $q(5)$, are generally concentrated within a narrower range than those of infant mortality, $q(1)$. The possible variability of the different estimates is illustrated in figure 14, in which the highest and lowest estimates associated with each age group of mother are plotted. The grey areas in the display represent, albeit roughly, the range of variation of possible estimates.

TABLE 16.   ESTIMATES OF INFANT AND UNDER-FIVE MORTALITY IN BANGLADESH, OBTAINED
USING THE COALE-DEMENY MORTALITY MODELS

Model	Age group of mother	Both sexes			Male			Female		
		Reference date	q(5)	q(1)	Reference date	q(5)	q(1)	Reference date	q(5)	q(1)
North	15-19	1973.1	.297	.177	1973.1	.304	.186	1973.1	.290	.167
	20-24	1971.7	.254	.151	1971.7	.261	.158	1971.8	.248	.142
	25-29	1969.8	.228	.135	1969.8	.238	.145	1969.8	.217	.125
	30-34	1967.6	.221	.131	1967.6	.229	.139	1967.6	.213	.122
	35-39	1965.1	.214	.127	1965.2	.221	.135	1965.1	.207	.119
	40-44	1962.5	.218	.129	1962.6	.221	.135	1962.4	.214	.123
	45-49	1959.7	.215	.127	1959.7	.212	.130	1959.6	.218	.125
South	15-19	1973.1	.294	.170	1973.1	.301	.179	1973.1	.280	.161
	20-24	1971.7	.248	.149	1971.7	.256	.157	1971.7	.240	.141
	25-29	1969.7	.230	.141	1969.7	.241	.150	1969.7	.218	.131
	30-34	1967.3	.230	.141	1967.4	.238	.149	1967.3	.221	.133
	35-39	1964.7	.229	.140	1964.8	.236	.147	1964.6	.222	.133
	40-44	1961.9	.237	.144	1962.0	.240	.150	1961.8	.234	.138
	45-49	1958.8	.239	.145	1958.9	.236	.148	1958.7	.243	.142
East	15-19	1973.1	.254	.187	1973.1	.261	.197	1973.1	.248	.176
	20-24	1971.6	.235	.174	1971.6	.242	.183	1971.7	.229	.164
	25-29	1969.6	.225	.167	1969.6	.235	.178	1969.6	.214	.154
	30-34	1967.2	.228	.169	1967.2	.235	.179	1967.1	.219	.158
	35-39	1964.5	.228	.169	1964.6	.235	.178	1964.4	.221	.159
	40-44	1961.6	.238	.176	1961.7	.241	.183	1961.5	.234	.167
	45-49	1958.4	.241	.178	1958.5	.238	.180	1958.3	.244	.174
West	15-19	1973.1	.273	.182	1973.1	.279	.192	1973.1	.266	.172
	20-24	1971.7	.244	.163	1971.7	.250	.172	1971.7	.237	.153
	25-29	1969.6	.228	.152	1969.7	.238	.164	1969.6	.217	.140
	30-34	1967.3	.227	.152	1967.3	.235	.161	1967.2	.218	.141
	35-39	1964.7	.224	.150	1964.8	.231	.159	1964.6	.216	.140
	40-44	1962.0	.230	.154	1962.1	.234	.161	1961.9	.226	.146
	45-49	1959.1	.229	.153	1959.2	.227	.156	1959.0	.230	.149

Model	Age group of mother	Both sexes			Male			Female		
		Reference date	$q(5)$	$q(1)$	Reference date	$q(5)$	$q(1)$	Reference date	$q(5)$	$q(1)$
Latin American	15-19	1973.2	.316	.179	1973.2	.307	.189	1973.2	[a]	[a]
	20-24	1971.8	.266	.155	1971.8	.268	.167	1971.8	.264	.142
	25-29	1970.0	.239	.142	1970.0	.248	.157	1970.0	.229	.127
	30-34	1967.8	.231	.138	1967.9	.239	.152	1967.8	.223	.124
	35-39	1965.4	.226	.135	1965.5	.232	.148	1965.3	.218	.122
	40-44	1962.6	.227	.136	1962.7	.230	.147	1962.5	.223	.124
	45-49	1959.0	.232	.138	1959.1	.230	.146	1958.9	.235	.129
Chilean	15-19	1973.0	.268	.199	1973.0	.272	.210	1973.0	.262	.188
	20-24	1971.7	.245	.185	1971.7	.251	.196	1971.7	.239	.174
	25-29	1969.8	.232	.176	1969.8	.242	.189	1969.8	.220	.162
	30-34	1967.5	.231	.175	1967.6	.239	.187	1967.5	.223	.164
	35-39	1965.0	.229	.174	1965.1	.235	.184	1964.9	.223	.164
	40-44	1962.2	.237	.179	1962.3	.240	.188	1962.1	.235	.171
	45-49	1958.6	.238	.180	1958.7	.235	.184	1958.5	.241	.175
South Asian	15-19	1973.2	.304	.179	1973.2	.311	.188	1973.2	.296	.169
	20-24	1971.8	.261	.157	1971.8	.268	.166	1971.8	.253	.149
	25-29	1969.9	.238	.146	1969.9	.249	.155	1969.9	.226	.136
	30-34	1967.7	.234	.143	1967.8	.241	.151	1967.7	.225	.136
	35-39	1965.2	.231	.142	1965.3	.237	.149	1965.1	.225	.135
	40-44	1962.3	.242	.148	1962.4	.244	.153	1962.2	.240	.143
	45-49	1958.4	.248	.151	1958.5	.245	.153	1958.3	.251	.148
Far Eastern	15-19	1973.1	.304	.183	1973.1	.325	.193	1973.1	.284	.172
	20-24	1971.7	.260	.160	1971.7	.271	.166	1971.7	.249	.155
	25-29	1969.9	.236	.148	1969.9	.247	.160	1969.9	.225	.136
	30-34	1967.7	.227	.144	1967.8	.235	.153	1967.7	.219	.134
	35-39	1965.3	.218	.139	1965.4	.223	.146	1965.3	.213	.131
	40-44	1962.7	.218	.139	1962.8	.219	.144	1962.6	.218	.133
	45-49	1959.4	.210	.134	1959.5	.209	.138	1959.3	.212	.130
General	15-19	1973.2	.302	.181	1973.2	.297	.191	1973.2	.286	.171
	20-24	1971.8	.261	.160	1971.8	.263	.172	1971.8	.259	.147
	25-29	1970.0	.237	.147	1970.0	.246	.162	1970.0	.227	.132
	30-34	1967.8	.229	.143	1967.8	.237	.157	1967.8	.221	.130
	35-39	1965.4	.223	.140	1965.4	.231	.153	1965.3	.216	.127
	40-44	1962.6	.224	.141	1962.7	.228	.152	1962.5	.220	.129
	45-49	1959.1	.226	.142	1959.2	.228	.152	1959.0	.227	.132

[a] Not available.

Figure 14 illustrates an important point: no matter which mortality model is chosen in applying the Brass estimation method, the errors that may affect the resulting estimates of $q(5)$ are likely to be smaller in both absolute and relative terms than those affecting $q(1)$. To give an example, suppose that the Chilean model is chosen to estimate mortality in childhood in Bangladesh, instead of the South or South Asian model. Then, considering only the most reliable estimates—those associated with age groups 25-29 to 35-39—one would obtain an estimate of $q(5)$ for both sexes combined close to .231 and a $q(1)$ of approximately .175, instead of the .230 and .141 values yielded by model South. If the South estimates are indeed correct, then the Chilean model will still estimate $q(5)$ fairly accurately but will overestimate $q(1)$ by some .034 points, or 24 per cent. At the other extreme, if model North were selected, $q(5)$ would be about .221 and $q(1)$ about .131, so that although both values would underestimate the South values by some .009 or .010 points, the error in $q(5)$ would be 4 per cent, as opposed to 7 per cent in $q(1)$.

These examples demonstrate the relative "robustness" of $q(5)$ as an indicator of mortality in childhood when it is estimated by the Brass method. An estimate is said to be robust when its value is not severely affected by deviations from the assumptions on which it is based. For the Brass method, $q(5)$ is more robust to the choice of mortality model than $q(1)$. This observation allows us to provide a partial answer to the question posed at the beginning of this section. The immediate consequence of choosing the wrong model is that the estimates obtained of under-five mortality will be biased. However, so long as only $q(5)$ is used as the common index, the magnitude of those biases is likely to be small, particularly for age groups above 20-24. If a different common index is opted for, robustness may decline. In particular, estimates of infant mortality, a very popular indicator, are especially sensitive to the choice of model and may be severely biased when the model used deviates markedly from the mortality pattern actually prevalent in the population under study.

In conclusion, if reliable evidence allowing an educated

Figure 12. Infant and under-five mortality for both sexes in Bangladesh,
estimated using the four Coale-Demeny mortality models

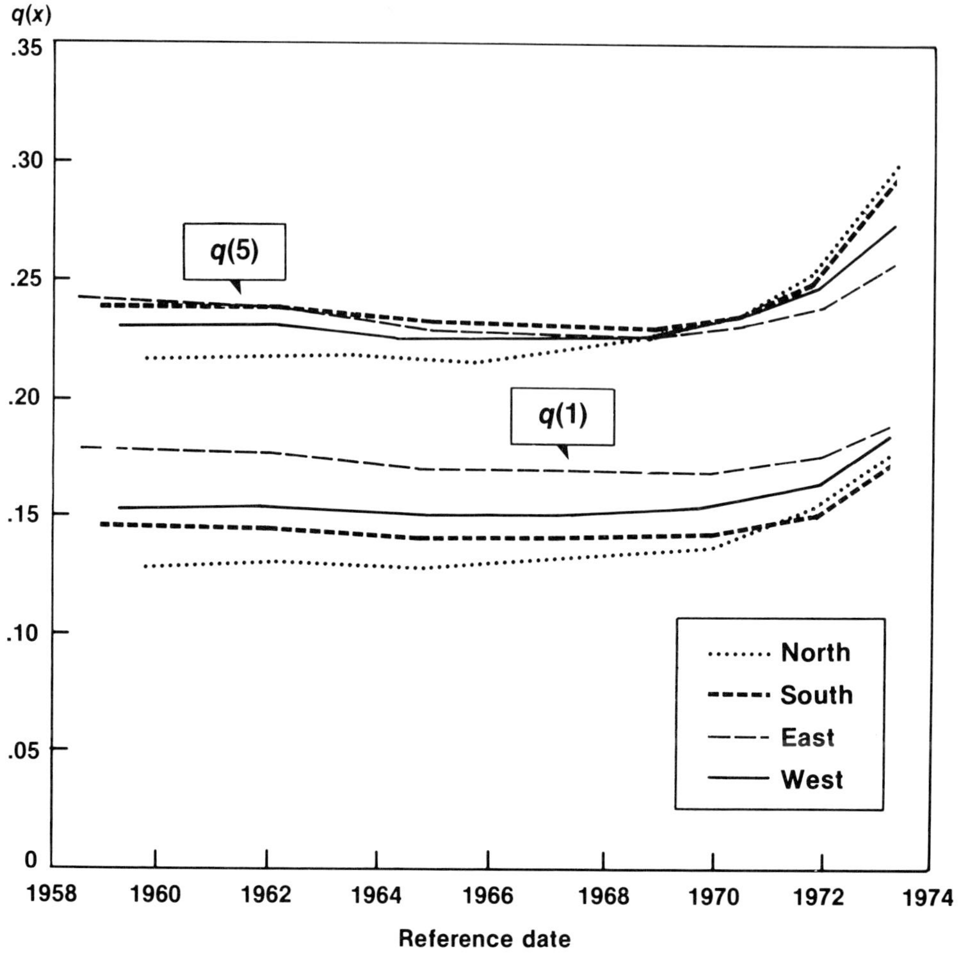

Source: Table 16.

choice of mortality model is lacking, errors in the estimates obtained are likely to result. Such errors, however, may be minimized by using $q(5)$ as a common index, as has been suggested in previous chapters of this *Guide*.

ANALYSIS OF DATA FROM SUCCESSIVE CENSUSES OR SURVEYS

In this section, the cases of two countries having more than one source of data on children ever born and surviving are discussed, in order to provide the reader with some guidance on how to evaluate and use the estimates obtained.

The first example is the case of Tunisia, whose 1966 and 1975 censuses gathered the information necessary to apply the Brass method. Table 18 presents the basic data and the estimates of under-five mortality obtained by using the Trussell version with model West. The estimated $q(5)$ values are plotted in figure 15. The most striking feature of those estimates is the declining trend they display. Since the estimates derived from the reports of younger women (mainly age group 15-19) are clearly biased upward, they should be disregarded.

Another noteworthy feature of the estimates for Tunisia is the high degree of consistency noticeable in the estimates derived from the reports of older women (aged 45-49) in 1975 (yielding an estimated $q(5)$ of .240 for early 1963) and those obtained from the reports of women aged 25-29 in 1966 (producing a $q(5)$ estimate of .245 for mid-1962). Such consistency is responsible for the relative smoothness of the trend suggested by the two curves in figure 15. Tunisia is thus a fairly exceptional case, in which the high consistency of the estimates derived from independent sources allows the analyst to adopt them at face value as indicators of the evolution of mortality in childhood. That is, disregarding the $q(5)$ estimates associated with younger age groups of women (15-19 and 20-24), it can be concluded that under-five mortality in Tunisia declined from 283 deaths per 1,000 births in late 1951 to 245 deaths per 1,000 births in the early 1960s, reaching a level of about 192 deaths per 1,000 births in early 1972.

The second example is provided by the case of Ecuador, where data on children ever born and surviving are available from three sources: the 1974 and 1982 censuses and the 1979 National Fertility Survey carried out as part of the World Fertility Survey programme. Table 19 presents the data available and the estimates they yield

50

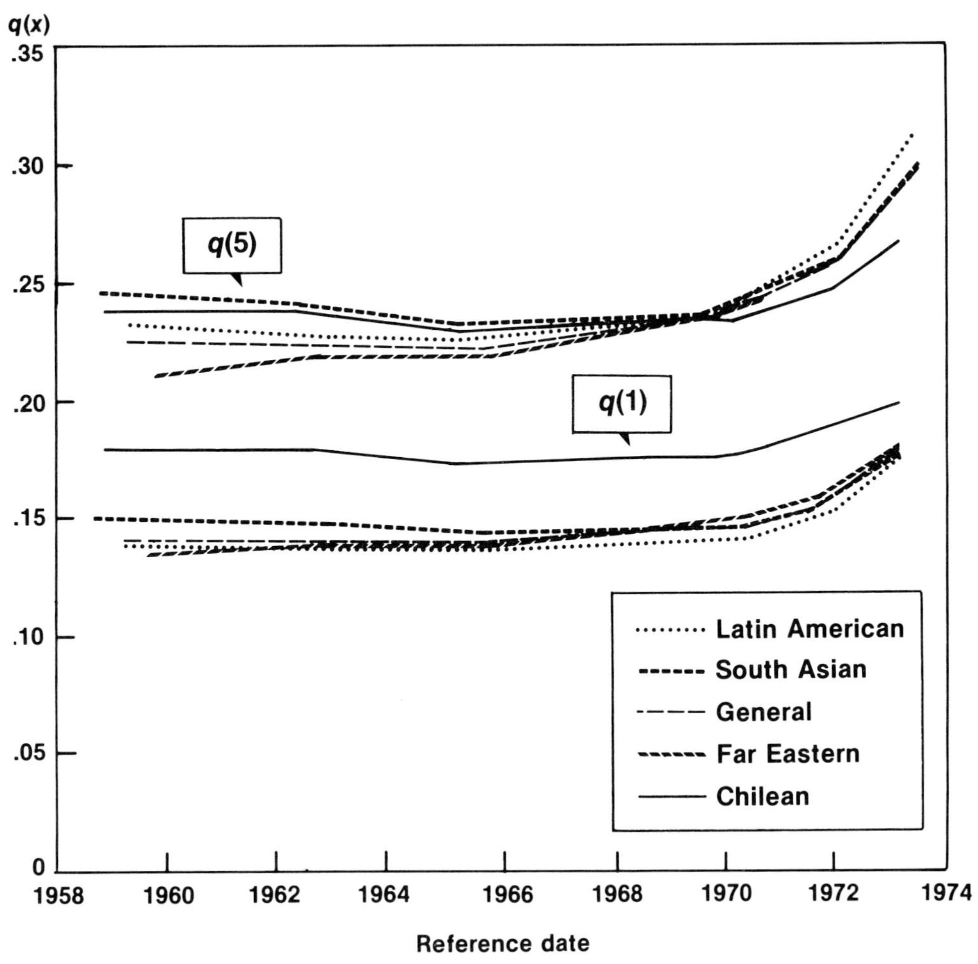

Figure 13. **Infant and under-five mortality for both sexes in Bangladesh, estimated using the five United Nations mortality models**

Source: Table 17.

TABLE 18. ESTIMATION OF UNDER-FIVE MORTALITY IN TUNISIA FROM DATA FROM SUCCESSIVE CENSUSES, USING MODEL WEST AND THE TRUSSELL VERSION OF THE BRASS METHOD

Age of mother	Number of women	Children ever born	Children surviving	Reference date	Estimated q(5)
		1966 census			
15-19	188 751	28 716	24 212	1965.5	.275
20-24	151 018	205 527	165 738	1964.3	.250
25-29	154 431	485 203	377 961	1962.4	.245
30-34	147 782	701 786	532 099	1960.1	.245
35-39	130 005	763 285	560 830	1957.5	.252
40-44	99 455	639 682	444 159	1954.7	.271
45-49	83 371	544 345	357 875	1951.7	.283
		1975 census			
15-19	307 400	11 620	9 800	1974.5	.282
20-24	244 010	168 780	145 010	1973.7	.193
25-29	168 800	425 400	355 750	1972.3	.192
30-34	136 650	578 450	471 590	1970.6	.197
35-39	151 910	852 160	674 140	1968.6	.208
40-44	135 830	908 660	686 760	1966.2	.227
45-49	113 030	796 250	573 820	1963.1	.240

Note: The census dates were 3 May 1966 and 8 May 1975.

Sources: Tunisia, Ministère du plan, Institut national de la statistique, *Recensement général de la population et des logements du 3 mai 1966*, vol. I, tables 17, 27 and 28; unpublished tables from the 8 May 1975 census.

Figure 14. **Range of variation of the possible estimates of infant and under-five mortality for both sexes in Bangladesh**

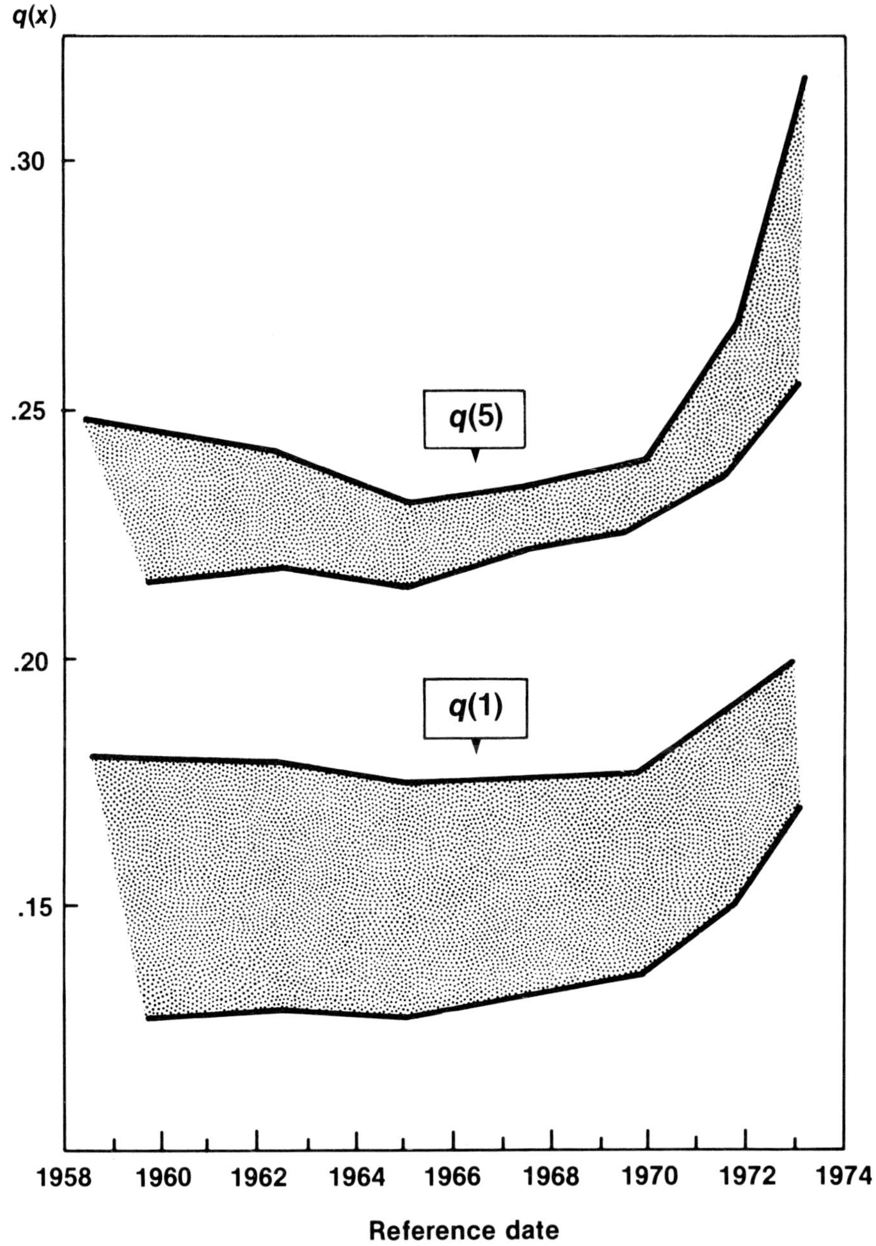

Source: Tables 16 and 17.

when model West is used. The different sets of estimates are displayed graphically in figure 16.

Note that, for Ecuador, the estimates obtained from different sources cover overlapping periods and are therefore more directly comparable with one another. As figure 16 shows, there is relatively good agreement between the estimates derived from the 1979 National Fertility Survey (from women in age groups 25-29 to 35-39) and those obtained from the 1982 census (from women in age groups 30-34 to 40-44). The 1974 census estimates covering the same period are noticeably higher, but some are derived from younger women (age groups 15-19 and 20-24) and may be biased upward. For earlier periods (1965-1968), the 1974 census estimates are directly comparable with those obtained from the reports of older women in 1979 (age groups 40-44 and 45-49). The latter, however, may be biased downward because of the omission of dead children that tends to affect the reports of older women. Therefore, the noticeable difference between the 1974 census estimates obtained from women in age groups 30-34 and 35-39 and those derived from women in age groups 40-44 and 45-49 at the time of the 1979 survey does not invalidate the former.

It is noteworthy that in Ecuador the degree of upward bias affecting the estimates derived from the reports of younger women is minor. In fact, for the 1982 census it is hardly noticeable, though this outcome may be the

Figure 15. Under-five mortality for both sexes in Tunisia, estimated using model West and the Trussell version of the Brass method

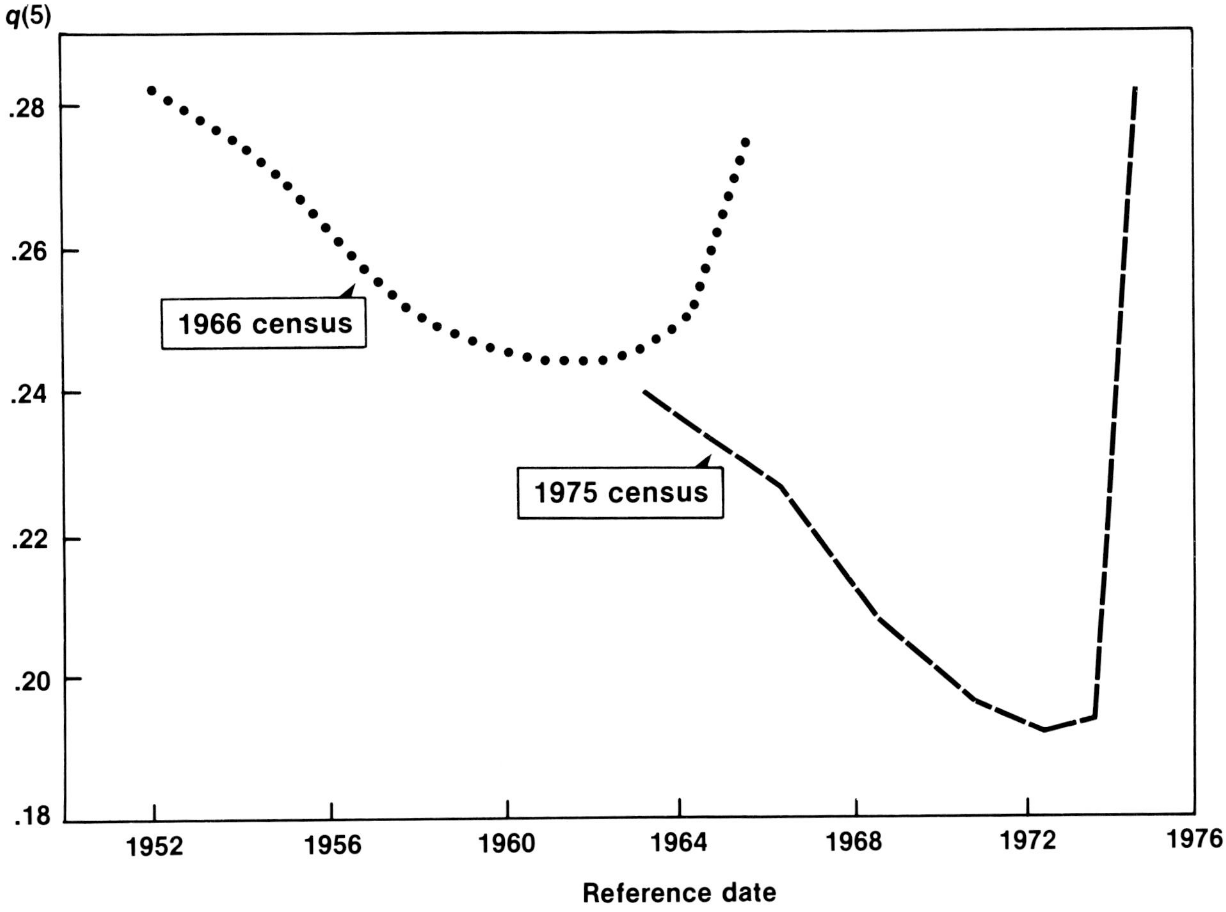

Source: Table 18

result of preliminary adjustments to the data (see table 19).

Although the estimates for Ecuador display considerably less consistency than those obtained in the case of Tunisia, it is still possible to infer from them the likely trend that mortality in childhood has followed through time. Estimates that could be used to determine that trend include the 1974 census estimates derived from age groups 30-34 to 40-44, the 1979 National Fertility Survey estimates derived from age groups 25-29 to 35-39 and the 1982 census estimates derived from age groups 25-29 and 30-34. The trend determined by those estimates implies that under-five mortality in Ecuador declined from about 173 deaths per 1,000 births in late 1962 to some 103 deaths per 1,000 births in mid-1978.

OVERALL OBSERVATIONS ON THE USE OF THE BRASS METHOD

To sum up, the five chapters describing the nature of the Brass method, the latest procedures available for its application and the problems faced in making use of those procedures and in using or interpreting the estimates obtained highlight the following features of the methodology as it now exists.

First, in populations for which reliable information about the prevalent pattern of mortality in childhood is lacking, there is always uncertainty about which mortality model to use in applying the Brass method. Although the use of $q(5)$—under-five mortality—as a common index reduces possible biases in the estimates obtained, they cannot be guaranteed to be accurate.

Second, the availability of a variety of mortality models gives the Brass method flexibility dealing with cases where independent evidence on the mortality pattern of the population involved can be obtained.

Third, given the upward biases that usually affect the estimates derived from the reports of younger women, estimates referring to recent periods usually have to be rejected as inaccurate. Thus, the most reliable estimates produced by the Brass method usually refer to a period between three and ten years preceding the time of interview, which limits their usefulness for the timely evaluation of the effects of health or development programmes.

Fourth, the power of the Brass method is increased when it can be applied to several data sets referring to the same population. The availability of independent estimates covering overlapping periods allows the analyst to

53

TABLE 19. ESTIMATION OF UNDER-FIVE MORTALITY IN ECUADOR FROM DATA FROM SEVERAL SOURCES, USING MODEL WEST AND THE TRUSSELL VERSION OF THE BRASS METHOD

Age of mother	Number of women	Children ever born	Children surviving	Reference date	Estimated $q(5)$
1974 census					
15-19	353 781	58 368	52 040	1973.5	.177
20-24	295 702	354 693	309 499	1972.2	.160
25-29	225 738	605 308	518 758	1970.4	.157
30-34	180 190	746 534	628 909	1968.1	.160
35-39	164 258	884 760	729 996	1965.6	.165
40-44	139 074	853 736	686 136	1962.9	.173
45-49	109 861	700 675	547 994	1959.9	.176
1979 National Fertility Survey					
15-19	1 680	288	262	1978.8	.142
20-24	1 377	1 585	1 422	1977.5	.127
25-29	1 074	2 672	2 364	1975.6	.125
30-34	883	3 568	3 084	1973.3	.137
35-39	717	3 913	3 350	1970.8	.135
40-44	586	3 728	3 078	1968.0	.153
45-49	480	3 255	2 624	1965.1	.156
1982 census[a]					
15-19	440 255	87 940	82 995	1981.8	.077
20-24	394 682	442 309	412 349	1980.5	.081
25-29	316 908	750 573	679 249	1978.6	.103
30-34	252 622	898 869	799 253	1976.4	.112
35-39	204 310	955 762	826 430	1974.0	.128
40-44	168 940	965 187	815 408	1971.4	.136
45-49	137 524	861 021	716 214	1968.5	.135

Note: The census dates were 8 June 1974 and 28 November 1982. The reference date for the National Fertility Survey was taken to be 1979.75.

[a]Preliminary data. The number of children surviving declared by women aged 15-19 has been adjusted.

Source: Ecuador, Ministerio de Salud Pública, *Encuesta Nacional de Salud Materno Infantil y Variables Demográficas—Ecuador 1982, Informe Final,* Tomo II (Quito, 1984), pp. 65 and 93-94.

Figure 16. Under-five mortality for both sexes in Ecuador, estimated using model West and the Trussell version of the Brass method

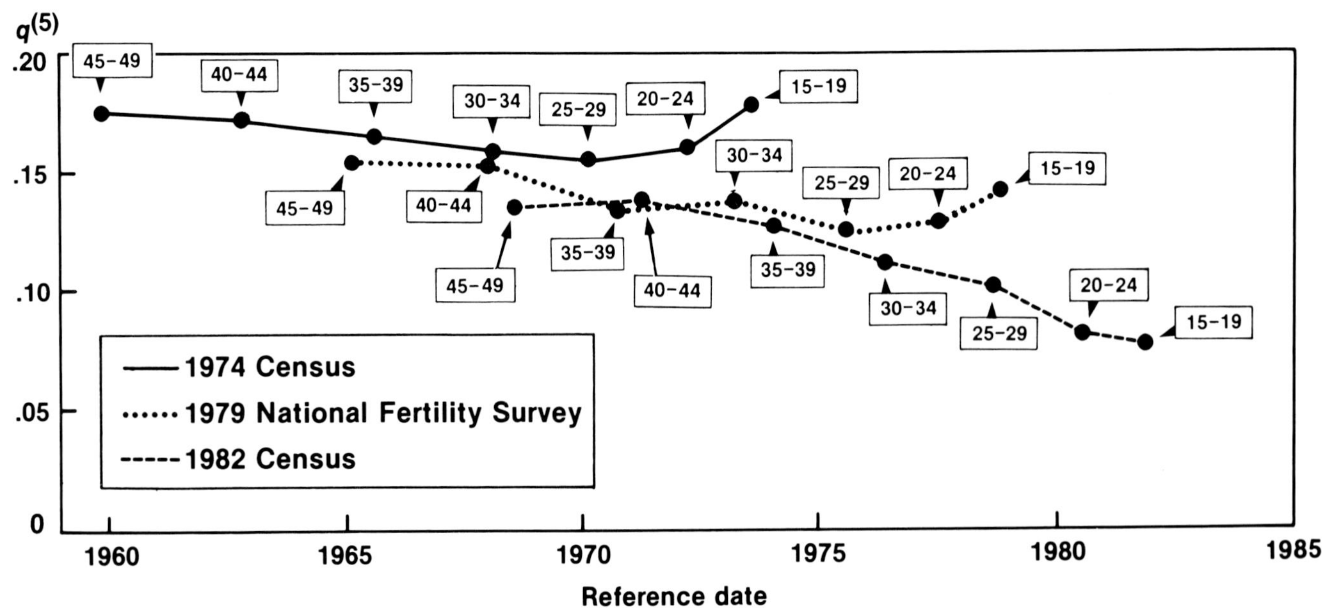

Source: Table 19.

check their consistency and select those less likely to be affected by extraneous biases.

These observations underscore both the strengths and the limitations of the Brass method. They do not reflect, however, the successful record that the method has had in allowing the estimation of mortality in childhood in populations with poor or defective data sources. During the more than twenty years of its existence, the Brass method has been instrumental in permitting, for the first time in history, a world-wide assessment of levels and trends of the mortality of children (see United Nations, 1988, and Bucht, 1988).

Chapter VII

BRASS-MACRAE METHOD

This chapter describes a method proposed only recently by W. Brass and S. Macrae (1984) to estimate mortality in childhood. The Brass-Macrae method is in some ways complementary to the original Brass method. It has the advantage of producing estimates for recent periods (about two years before the time of interview) and is based on data that may be collected at relatively low cost. Its main drawback is that the data it uses may not be representative. Indeed, since the Brass-Macrae procedure envisages that only women about to give birth will be asked about the survivorship of their previous child, the children whose mortality is being measured may not be representative of all children. In cases where only women giving birth in hospitals or in government clinics are interviewed, the data will be even less representative of the total population. Strategies to make the data used more representative and efforts to understand the possible biases to which they are subject or to devise means of eliminating such biases are currently being pursued.[3] Yet, it is likely that those efforts may result in a considerably more complex estimation procedure than the one presented in this *Guide*.

Simplicity is an important advantage of the Brass-Macrae method, and thus may be worth maintaining even at the expense of full representativeness or perfect accuracy of the data. So far, the method has been largely applied to data gathered in specific areas—a given town or city or even a given hospital.[4] Consequently, it has been clear from the start that the population under study was not representative of the whole population of a country. In certain circumstances, nationally representative data may not be required, as, for instance, when a programme to improve child nutrition operates only in a given region. In such cases, the Brass-Macrae method may be used by programme managers to monitor changes in child mortality only in the region of interest. It can also be argued that, for purposes of monitoring change, biases affecting the Brass-Macrae estimates may be discounted as long as they remain constant. The researcher must, however, be aware of the possible sources of bias, in order to be able to ascertain the likelihood of biases remaining constant through time.

Owing to its recency, the Brass-Macrae method is still in the process of being tested. Several organizations, including UNICEF, the Latin American Demographic Centre (CELADE) and the London School of Hygiene and Tropical Medicine, are currently engaged in experimental applications of the method and are trying to determine how best to gather the basic information needed for its use.[5] Although the method seems promising, it is still difficult to judge its efficacy or to evaluate its performance under a variety of circumstances. Hence, the conclusions presented in this chapter are necessarily tentative and may err on the side of caution.

NATURE OF THE BASIC DATA

The Brass-Macrae method derives measures of child mortality from information obtained at or near the birth of a child about the survival of the mother's previous child (and sometimes about the child born prior to that one also). Unlike the Brass method, the information used in applying the Brass-Macrae method is derived from administrative sources (such as health-centre records) rather than from population censuses or surveys. The additional costs of data collection are thus small, since all that is generally required is the addition of two or three questions to an existing administrative form. The questions could be:

1. Have you been pregnant before?   Yes/No

2. If yes: Was the child of your previous pregnancy born alive?   Yes/No

3. If yes: Is that child still alive?   Yes/No

An advantage of these questions is that they require very simple answers that do not even involve numbers. In that respect, they are likely to elicit more reliable information than the questions used to gather the data required for the Brass method.

As already mentioned, the Brass-Macrae method uses data that do not necessarily reflect the mortality experience of all children in a given population. In particular, deaths among the last-born children of all women in the population remain unrecorded. Also, because women are interviewed only at the time they give birth, the experience of the highly fecund is more likely to be recorded. Biases arising from such selectivity will always be in operation, even if all women giving birth in a country are interviewed. However, there is reason to believe that in populations where fertility is still moderate to high, the resulting biases would be minimal.

In general, it is not expected that the data necessary for the application of the Brass-Macrae method would be obtained from a nationally representative sample. A hospital or clinic is the typical setting envisaged for the collection of the basic information, although it has been suggested that midwives aiding in home deliveries might be trained to gather the necessary data. Such an approach to data collection would be mandatory in countries or regions where a majority of women give birth at home. Although nationally representative data may not be necessary for monitoring and evaluating local interventions aimed at reducing mortality, it is still important to define the target population and take steps to ensure that the data gathered are in effect representative of that population.

DERIVATION OF THE METHOD AND ITS RATIONALE

It is easy to understand intuitively how the method works. Let us assume that all live-birth intervals are 2.5 years long and that every woman is asked at the time of delivery whether she has previously given birth and, if so, whether the previous-born child is still alive. Then, each previous child will have been exposed to the risk of dying for exactly 2.5 years, and the proportion dead will equal the cohort probability of dying by age 2.5, $q(2.5)$, provided that all last-born children have the same mortality experience as children whose birth is followed by that of a sibling.

In practice, of course, birth intervals are not all exactly 2.5 years long, though almost all are within the range of one to five years. Thus, the proportion dead of previous children represents a weighted average of the probabilities of dying between birth and ages 1-5 for cohorts born between one and five years before interview, the weights being the proportions of women having each length of birth interval.

Using models of birth intervals and mortality in childhood, Brass and Macrae found that the proportion dead of previous children is, in most high-fertility populations, a close approximation to the probability of dying by exact age 2, $q(2)$, and that the proportion dead of next-to-previous children is a close approximation to the probability of dying by exact age 5, $q(5)$. Since the proportions dead are strongly influenced by the age pattern of mortality in childhood—that is, most child deaths occur at very early ages—the $q(x)$ estimates obtained from them are reasonably robust to variations in birth-interval distributions. Adjustments can be made for the effects of such variations if the necessary information on average birth-interval lengths is available.

Brass and Macrae found that the proportion dead of previous children approximates $q(0.8z)$, where z is the length in years of the average birth interval. For average birth intervals of 30 months (2.5 years), the proportion dead corresponds to $q(2)$. Because the distribution of birth intervals by length varies little with respect to fertility level, the method is not overly sensitive to changes in fertility, especially because fertility declines are mainly due to a reduction of completed family size rather than to the substantial lengthening of birth intervals.

The estimates of $q(2)$ and $q(5)$ yielded by the Brass-Macrae method refer to different birth cohorts and may be equated to period estimates provided that some allowance is made for the timing of deaths. Aguirre and Hill (1987) have estimated, on the basis of declared dates of birth and death for previous and next-to-previous children, that $q(2)$ refers to a point approximately two years preceding interview and $q(5)$ refers to a point between three and four years preceding interview. Although those estimates of timing refer to a particular case, they provide a good indication of the rough reference dates of the $q(x)$ estimates obtained.

LIMITATIONS OF THE BRASS-MACRAE METHOD

Because of the data it uses and the simplifying assumptions made in its application, the Brass-Macrae method has certain limitations, which are discussed in some detail below.

First, the data used exclude information on all last-born children. Such exclusion is not serious in high-fertility populations, but in those populations where completed family size is small (two or three children per woman), a large proportion of first-born children will be included in the data used for estimation purposes, and their mortality experience may not be representative of average mortality levels in the total population of children. However, in contrast with the Brass method, the Brass-Macrae approach is based on data on recent births of all orders to women of all ages and is therefore less likely to display the biases associated with the increased mortality of children whose mothers are very young.

Secondly, the Brass-Macrae method as described below makes no explicit allowance for changing fertility and mortality conditions. Fertility declines due to significant increases in average birth intervals will lead to overestimates of mortality when the proportion dead of previous children is simply equated to $q(2)$. Mortality declines, on the other hand, will start to be reflected in the $q(2)$ estimates only two or three years after they occur and will be fully reflected in those estimates only five years after their inception. Thus, as with the Brass method, sharp declines in mortality will appear as a smoothed downward curve, but, in contrast with the Brass method, the downward trend will not pre-date the inception of mortality change.

Thirdly, a single application of the Brass-Macrae method does not allow the estimation of trends in child mortality. Data relating to several years of observation are required to obtain some indication of trends.

Fourthly, since the Brass-Macrae method does not rely on data obtained through surveys based on probabilistic samples, the estimates it yields often do not refer to the total population of a country or even of a region. Biases due to the selectivity of the population under consideration (that using health clinics, for example) are likely to affect the estimates obtained and should be taken into account by the analyst in making comparison with estimates yielded by other methods.

APPLICATION OF THE BRASS-MACRAE METHOD

Data required

The Brass-Macrae method estimates probabilities of dying in childhood from proportions dead of previous and, if data are available, next-to-previous children, the information being collected from women at or just after the birth of the most recent child.

Hence, the only data required are the following:

1. The number of women giving birth who reported having had a previous child, irrespective of their age, marital status etc.;

2. The number of women giving birth who, having had a previous child, reported that that child had died.

If questions on the survival of the next-to-previous child are also posed, then the following will also be needed:

3. The number of women giving birth who reported having had a child before the previous one;

4. The number of women giving birth who, having had a child before the previous one, reported that that child had died.

Note that there is no need for information on the number of children ever born or the total number of women. The data needed can be easily collected at the time of delivery, and it is not strictly necessary to compile a year's worth of data to apply the method. Since any seasonal variation in child mortality will be largely smoothed out by variability in birth intervals, as long as a sufficient number of events are recorded, there is no minimum length of time for which the data-collection exercise must be maintained. As noted earlier, however, data collection must be maintained over a period of years to estimate trends in child mortality.

Computational procedure

The computational procedure is very simple, consisting of, at most, two steps.

Step 1. *Calculation of the probabilities of dying,* q*(2) and* q*(5)*

The probability of dying by age 2, $q(2)$, is calculated by dividing the number of women reporting a previous child who has died by the total number of women reporting a previous child. Thus,

$$q^e(2) = \frac{NPCD(1)}{NPC(1)} \qquad (7.1)$$

where $q^e(2)$ is the estimated probability of dying by age 2, $NPCD(1)$ is the number of women with a previous child dead, and $NPC(1)$ is the number of women who reported a previous child. Cases of non-response, where the mother does not report the survival status of the child, should be excluded from both the numerator and the denominator.

The probability of dying by age 5, $q(5)$, is similarly calculated by dividing the number of women reporting a next-to-previous child dead by the number of women reporting a next-to-previous child. Thus,

$$q^e(5) = \frac{NPCD(2)}{NPC(2)} \qquad (7.2)$$

where the symbols have the same meanings as before, but refer to next-to-previous rather than to previous births.

Step 2. *Conversion to a common index*

In cases where estimates of both $q(2)$ and $q(5)$ can be obtained, conversion to a common index is necessary to compare them. For consistency's sake, it is recommended that $q(5)$ be used as the common index, just as in the application of the Brass method. It is therefore necessary to find a value $q^c(5)$ equivalent to the $q^e(2)$ estimate obtained above. As with the Brass method, a model-life-table family must be used to perform the necessary conversion. Ideally, the family used should reflect the

mortality pattern prevalent in early childhood in the population being studied (see chapter I).

Having selected an appropriate model-life-table family from annex I or II, one needs to identify two mortality levels, j and $j + 1$, whose $q(2)$ values enclose the estimated $q^e(2)$ so that

$$q^j(2) > q^e(2) > q^{j+1}(2) \qquad (7.3)$$

The desired value of $q^c(5)$ is then obtained as

$$q^c(5) = (1.0 - h)q^j(5) + h\,q^{j+1}(5) \qquad (7.4)$$

where $q^j(5)$ and $q^{j+1}(5)$ are the model values of $q(5)$ at levels j and $j + 1$, respectively, in the selected family of model life tables, and h is an interpolation factor calculated as follows:

$$h = \frac{q^e(2) - q^j(2)}{q^{j+1}(2) - q^j(2)} \qquad (7.5)$$

Once $q^c(5)$ is calculated, it can be compared with the $q^e(5)$ obtained in step 1. Since the latter refers to a slightly earlier period than $q^c(5)$, under conditions of declining mortality $q^c(5)$ should be lower than $q^e(5)$. The example presented below illustrates such a comparison.

A detailed example

The data for this detailed example were collected in five health facilities in Bamako, Mali, starting in January 1985 (Hill and others, 1985). A specially designed form was used to gather information about all deliveries and the previous two live births that each mother might have had. Table 20 shows the number of previous births and next-to-previous births recorded, and the number of children who had died by the time of observation.

TABLE 20.   ESTIMATION OF THE PROBABILITY OF DYING $q(x)$,
FOR BAMAKO, MALI, USING THE BRASS-MACRAE METHOD

	Number of births (1)	Number dead (2)	Probability of dying (3)
Previous...........................	4 775	679	.1422
Next to previous.................	3 737	620	.1659

Source: A. G. Hill and others, "L'enquête pilote sur la mortalité aux jeunes âges dans cinq maternités de la ville de Bamako, Mali", in *Estimation de la mortalité du jeune enfant (0-5) pour guider les actions de santé dans les pays en développement*, Séminaire INSERM, vol. 145, (Paris, 1985), pp. 107-130.

Step 1. *Calculation of the probabilities of dying,* q*(2) and* q*(5)*

For each class of previous births, the probabilities of dying are calculated according to equations 7.1 and 7.2 by dividing the entries of column 2 of table 20 by those of column 1, as shown below:

$$q^e(2) = \frac{679}{4,775} = .1422$$

$$q^e(5) = \frac{620}{3,737} = .1659$$

The resulting $q^e(2)$ and $q^e(5)$ estimates are displayed in column 3 of table 20.

Step 2. *Conversion to a common index*

Using $q(5)$ as the common index, $q^e(2)$ needs to be converted into an equivalent measure of $q(5)$. For both sexes and a sex ratio at birth of 1.05 male births per female birth, the Coale-Demeny North model-life-table values in table A.I.9 show that the estimated $q^e(2)$ value is enclosed by $q^{13}(2) = .14701$, whose $q^{13}(5) = .19235$, and by $q^{14}(2) = .13158$, for which $q^{14}(5) = .17113$. Using equation 7.5 to estimate the interpolation factor h,

$$h = \frac{.14220 - .14701}{.13158 - .14701} = .3247$$

This value of h is then used in equation 7.4 to find the corresponding $q^c(5)$ as follows:

$$q^c(5) = (1.0 - .3247)(.19235) + (.3247)(.17113)$$

$$= .185$$

Note that this $q^c(5)$ value is considerably higher than the $q^e(5)$ value obtained in step 1, namely, .166. Such estimates would imply that under-five mortality among the children of interviewed women increased from .166 in 1981-1982 (three to four years before interview) to .185 around 1983 (about two years before interview). The unlikelihood of such an increase suggests that the estimates obtained may be subject to selection biases that affect their accuracy. Aguirre and Hill (1987) argue that $q^e(5)$ is more likely to be affected by those biases, since it is based on children whose mothers are older on average and who seem to represent only the better educated and socially advantaged group of the population (older Bamako women who have already had several children tend not to give birth in clinics). For that reason, $q^e(5)$ is lower than expected, and it would have to be rejected as a valid estimate of under-five mortality for 1981-1982. On the other hand, there is no reason to reject $q^c(5)$, which, at 185 deaths per 1,000 live births, would be an estimate of the 1983 probability of dying by age 5 among the children born to women who attended health clinics in Bamako.

COMMENTS ON THE RESULTS OF THE METHOD

As stated earlier, experience in the use of the Brass-Macrae method is limited, so no firm assertions can as yet be made about the validity of the estimates it provides. In the example presented above, the inconsistencies discovered should raise doubts about the accuracy of the estimates obtained. However Aguirre and Hill (1987) note that the estimated $q(2)$ value of .142 is in line with estimates obtained, using the original Brass method, from a large survey conducted by the Sahel Institute among a representative sample of Bamako households. Note that estimates obtained by applying the original Brass method are needed to validate the Brass-Macrae results. The assessment of new techniques in terms of the old is to be expected and will probably continue for a few years. For that reason, the reader should become familiar with both methods.

Mention has been made of the potential use of the Brass-Macrae method to assess trends in child mortality in specific subpopulations. Perhaps one of the best examples so far of that use is provided by the data gathered through the birth-notification scheme operating in Solomon Islands during the period 1968-1975 and analysed by Brass and Macrae in their 1984 article. Table 21 presents the basic data and the $q(2)$ estimates derived from them. Although for earlier years the $q(2)$ estimates vary in an unexpected fashion, the full set of estimates shows sustained mortality decline. Indeed, if the likely reference dates of the estimates are taken into account, mortality in childhood seems to have been cut almost in half between 1968 and 1975.

TABLE 21. ESTIMATION OF THE PROBABILITY OF DYING BY AGE 2, $q(2)$, FOR SOLOMON ISLANDS, USING THE BRASS-MACRAE METHOD

Year of notification	Number of previous births (1)	Number dead (2)	Probability of dying $q(2)$ (3)
1968	1 769	209	.1181
1969	2 400	255	.1063
1970	2 796	331	.1184
1971	3 030	281	.0927
1972	3 861	333	.0862
1973	3 369	228	.0677
1974	2 390	159	.0665
1975	4 472	264	.0590

Source: W. Brass and S. Macrae, "Childhood mortality estimated from reports on previous births given by mothers at the time of a maternity: I. Preceding-births technique", *Asian and Pacific Census Forum,* vol. 11, No. 2 (November 1984), p. 7.

By permitting the estimation of child mortality over a period of years, the data for Solomon Islands provide an example of a more realistic use of the Brass-Macrae technique than does the case of Mali. Even if the estimated $q(2)$ values are not perfect, their declining trend is indicative of the changes taking place and might serve as an adequate evaluation tool. It is important, however, to confirm that the representativeness of the basic data has remained constant through time, especially in view of the variability evident in the numbers of women providing information (see column 1 of table 21). Brass and Macrae noted that "some selection bias is likely since the births notified may be to women who are better educated or otherwise socially advantaged",[6] but they discounted the effects of that bias. The existence of such selectivity could be assessed by gathering additional information on the women giving birth, including their age, parity, educational level, work status and usual place of residence. The distribution of reporting women according to those variables would shed light on the likelihood and possible extent of biases stemming from changes in selectivity.

Clearly, because of its simplicity and flexibility, the Brass-Macrae method deserves attention. The tests it is being subjected to will, it is hoped, show that the selectivity and other biases that may affect the estimates it yields may reasonably be discounted by analysts

59

interested in assessing programme impact. It is unlikely, however, that the Brass-Macrae method will replace the original Brass method as the main technique providing national estimates of mortality in childhood. It is in providing estimates for selected subpopulations that the Brass-Macrae method has the greatest potential.

ANNEX I
Coale-Demeny model life table values for probabilities of dying
between birth and exact age x, $q(x)$

TABLES

		Page
A.I.1.	North model values for male probabilities of dying, $q(x)$	61
A.I.2.	South model values for male probabilities of dying, $q(x)$	62
A.I.3.	East model values for male probabilities of dying, $q(x)$	62
A.I.4.	West model values for male probabilities of dying, $q(x)$	63
A.I.5.	North model values for female probabilities of dying, $q(x)$	63
A.I.6.	South model values for female probabilities of dying, $q(x)$	64
A.I.7.	East model values for female probabilities of dying, $q(x)$	64
A.I.8.	West Asian model values for female probabilities of dying, $q(x)$	65
A.I.9.	North model values for probabilities of dying, $q(x)$, both sexes combined	65
A.I.10.	South model values for probabilities of dying, $q(x)$, both sexes combined	66
A.I.11.	East model values for probabilities of dying, $q(x)$, both sexes combined	66
A.I.12.	West model values for probabilities of dying, $q(x)$, both sexes combined	67

TABLE A.I.1.   NORTH MODEL VALUES FOR MALE PROBABILITIES OF DYING, $q(x)$

Level	e_0	$q(1)$	$q(2)$	$q(3)$	$q(5)$	$q(10)$	$q(15)$	$q(20)$
1	17.6	.37117	.45216	.50142	.56587	.62135	.64586	.66959
2	19.9	.33923	.41659	.46363	.52518	.58040	.60516	.62944
3	22.3	.31056	.38401	.42867	.48711	.54145	.56616	.59070
4	24.7	.28459	.35397	.39617	.45138	.50437	.52877	.55331
5	27.2	.26089	.32613	.36581	.41773	.46899	.49289	.51722
6	29.6	.23913	.30021	.33735	.38595	.43520	.45842	.48238
7	32.0	.21904	.27596	.31058	.35588	.40287	.42527	.44871
8	34.5	.20041	.25322	.28533	.32735	.37191	.39338	.41617
9	36.9	.18306	.23181	.26146	.30024	.34222	.36266	.38470
10	39.3	.16686	.21161	.23883	.27443	.31373	.33306	.35426
11	41.8	.15167	.19251	.21734	.24983	.28635	.30452	.32481
12	44.3	.13744	.17444	.19694	.22639	.26008	.27703	.29635
13	46.7	.12411	.15672	.17656	.20251	.23311	.24884	.26736
14	49.1	.11228	.14080	.15814	.18084	.20839	.22285	.24042
15	51.5	.10074	.12544	.14046	.16010	.18463	.19778	.21429
16	53.9	.08955	.10995	.12293	.14031	.16186	.17366	.18903
17	56.3	.07874	.09527	.10632	.12145	.14006	.15051	.16466
18	58.8	.06833	.08145	.09063	.10348	.11924	.12831	.14120
19	61.3	.05836	.06844	.07584	.08638	.09935	.10706	.11865
20	63.9	.04885	.05622	.06189	.07011	.08037	.08673	.09700
21	66.4	.03981	.04476	.04874	.05462	.06224	.06727	.07621
22	68.9	.03130	.03405	.03635	.03979	.04490	.04863	.05622
23	71.6	.02353	.02516	.02659	.02876	.03219	.03487	.04062
24	74.4	.01606	.01690	.01766	.01883	.02084	.02255	.02674
25	77.3	.01056	.01096	.01134	.01193	.01303	.01408	.01702

TABLE A.I.2.   SOUTH MODEL VALUES FOR MALE PROBABILITIES OF DYING, $q(x)$

Level	e_0	$q(1)$	$q(2)$	$q(3)$	$q(5)$	$q(10)$	$q(15)$	$q(20)$
1	19.9	.33555	.46045	.51806	.56599	.60074	.61600	.63801
2	22.3	.31122	.42918	.48359	.52885	.56317	.57843	.60052
3	24.7	.28925	.40024	.45143	.49402	.52756	.54267	.56461
4	27.0	.26924	.37330	.42131	.46124	.49374	.50857	.53016
5	29.3	.25089	.34813	.39298	.43029	.46154	.47599	.49707
6	31.6	.23396	.32449	.36625	.40099	.43083	.44480	.46525
7	33.9	.21828	.30224	.34097	.37319	.40148	.41491	.43460
8	36.2	.20368	.28122	.31699	.34674	.37339	.38622	.40507
9	38.5	.19004	.26132	.29420	.32155	.34647	.35865	.37659
10	40.6	.17752	.24318	.27346	.29866	.32152	.33299	.35007
11	42.9	.16642	.22532	.25249	.27510	.29600	.30675	.32276
12	45.1	.15559	.20812	.23235	.25251	.27145	.28147	.29637
13	47.4	.14502	.19155	.21300	.23086	.24786	.25711	.27086
14	49.6	.13475	.17558	.19442	.21099	.22518	.23364	.24261
15	51.9	.12478	.16022	.17657	.19017	.20338	.21104	.22242
16	54.1	.11513	.14545	.15944	.17107	.18242	.18928	.19946
17	56.3	.10581	.13125	.14299	.15275	.16228	.16833	.17730
18	58.6	.09676	.11733	.12693	.13502	.14275	.14798	.15574
19	61.2	.08618	.10112	.10835	.11472	.12079	.12520	.13164
20	63.7	.07610	.08735	.09300	.09817	.10291	.10655	.11186
21	66.1	.06605	.07420	.07845	.08248	.08604	.08896	.09320
22	68.5	.05605	.06167	.06472	.06770	.07024	.07251	.07575
23	71.0	.04617	.04980	.05184	.05391	.05561	.05727	.05962
24	73.6	.03648	.03863	.03988	.04118	.04223	.04336	.04494
25	76.0	.02822	.02943	.03016	.03094	.03155	.03229	.03332

TABLE A.I.3.   EAST MODEL VALUES FOR MALE PROBABILITIES OF DYING, $q(x)$

Level	e_0	$q(1)$	$q(2)$	$q(3)$	$q(5)$	$q(10)$	$q(15)$	$q(20)$
1	17.4	.50506	.57037	.59752	.62736	.65321	.66440	.68063
2	19.9	.46449	.52896	.55576	.58522	.61153	.62306	.63989
3	22.4	.42751	.49039	.51654	.54527	.57165	.58336	.60054
4	24.9	.39356	.45430	.47956	.50731	.53345	.54519	.56253
5	27.4	.36222	.42040	.44459	.47117	.49679	.50846	.52579
6	29.9	.33314	.38844	.41143	.43670	.46159	.47308	.49025
7	32.3	.30604	.35822	.37992	.40376	.42775	.43897	.45586
8	34.8	.28069	.32958	.34991	.37225	.39517	.40605	.42256
9	37.2	.25691	.30238	.32128	.34206	.36379	.37427	.39030
10	39.6	.23453	.27648	.29392	.31309	.33353	.34357	.35904
11	42.1	.21359	.25130	.26698	.28421	.30305	.31267	.32767
12	44.4	.19438	.22804	.24203	.25741	.27477	.28390	.29830
13	46.7	.17584	.20561	.21799	.23159	.24744	.25602	.26973
14	49.0	.15796	.18401	.19484	.20674	.22104	.22903	.24198
15	51.3	.14077	.16324	.17258	.18285	.19557	.20295	.21506
16	53.7	.12426	.14329	.15121	.15991	.17104	.17776	.18899
17	56.0	.10842	.12414	.13067	.13786	.14741	.15345	.16375
18	58.4	.09328	.10558	.11082	.11671	.12467	.13003	.13936
19	60.7	.07883	.08773	.09173	.09643	.10282	.10748	.11583
20	63.0	.06506	.07087	.07363	.07700	.08182	.08578	.09312
21	65.3	.05143	.05534	.05729	.05977	.06351	.06675	.07290
22	67.7	.03892	.04135	.04262	.04429	.04692	.04944	.05438
23	70.2	.02760	.02896	.02971	.03072	.03241	.03424	.03800
24	72.7	.01782	.01847	.01885	.01936	.02033	.02153	.02416
25	75.3	.01011	.01037	.01052	.01074	.01120	.01190	.01354

Level	e_0	$q(1)$	$q(2)$	$q(3)$	$q(5)$	$q(10)$	$q(15)$	$q(20)$
1	18.0	.41907	.49692	.53102	.56995	.59898	.61840	.64324
2	20.4	.38343	.45848	.49135	.52888	.55789	.57742	.60260
3	22.9	.35132	.42310	.45454	.49043	.51907	.53849	.56369
4	25.3	.32215	.39033	.42020	.45429	.48231	.50142	.52640
5	27.7	.29546	.35985	.38805	.42024	.44742	.46607	.49062
6	30.1	.27089	.33135	.35783	.38806	.41425	.43230	.45625
7	32.5	.24817	.30463	.32936	.35758	.38263	.40000	.42320
8	34.9	.22706	.27948	.30244	.32865	.35246	.36905	.39138
9	37.3	.20737	.25575	.27693	.30112	.32361	.33936	.36074
10	39.7	.18895	.23329	.25272	.27489	.29599	.31084	.33118
11	42.1	.17165	.21200	.22968	.24985	.26952	.28343	.30266
12	44.5	.15537	.19178	.20772	.22592	.24412	.25704	.27511
13	47.1	.13942	.17088	.18466	.20039	.21685	.22853	.24544
14	49.6	.12453	.15167	.16356	.17713	.19200	.20266	.21833
15	51.8	.11136	.13477	.14502	.15673	.17012	.17982	.19429
16	54.1	.09857	.11836	.12708	.13707	.14897	.15766	.17088
17	56.5	.08621	.10210	.10944	.11816	.12855	.13623	.14813
18	58.8	.07430	.08666	.09264	.09999	.10888	.11553	.12609
19	61.2	.06287	.07204	.07668	.08256	.08996	.09556	.10476
20	63.6	.05193	.05821	.06153	.06585	.07177	.07634	.08416
21	66.0	.04091	.04492	.04715	.05011	.05464	.05826	.06469
22	68.6	.03075	.03325	.03469	.03666	.03996	.04266	.04766
23	71.2	.02144	.02281	.02364	.02479	.02697	.02881	.03242
24	73.9	.01332	.01395	.01434	.01490	.01615	.01727	.01959
25	76.6	.00711	.00734	.00748	.00769	.00829	.00886	.01015

Level	e_0	$q(1)$	$q(2)$	$q(3)$	$q(5)$	$q(10)$	$q(15)$	$q(20)$
1	20.0	.31973	.40293	.45415	.52217	.58336	.61121	.63767
2	22.5	.29202	.37069	.41911	.48342	.54353	.57130	.59794
3	25.0	.26715	.34121	.38680	.44735	.50584	.53325	.55977
4	27.5	.24461	.31408	.35684	.41363	.47010	.49691	.52307
5	30.0	.22405	.28896	.32892	.38199	.43613	.46215	.48775
6	32.5	.20517	.26560	.30280	.35220	.40378	.42885	.45374
7	35.0	.18774	.24378	.27827	.32408	.37292	.39692	.42095
8	37.5	.17158	.22332	.25517	.29747	.34343	.36627	.38933
9	40.0	.15653	.20409	.23336	.27223	.31521	.33680	.35880
10	42.5	.14247	.18595	.21271	.24825	.28818	.30846	.32932
11	45.0	.12930	.16881	.19313	.22543	.26225	.28117	.30083
12	47.5	.11695	.15261	.17456	.20372	.23741	.25493	.27334
13	50.0	.10549	.13681	.15609	.18169	.21178	.22788	.24517
14	52.5	.09502	.12190	.13860	.16094	.18739	.20191	.21784
15	55.0	.08488	.10753	.12187	.14136	.16436	.17730	.19180
16	57.5	.07508	.09395	.10612	.12290	.14264	.15401	.16705
17	60.0	.06565	.08113	.09129	.10550	.12213	.13197	.14354
18	62.5	.05663	.06904	.07733	.08907	.10276	.11110	.12121
19	65.0	.04801	.05764	.06417	.07355	.08444	.09132	.09996
20	67.5	.03982	.04689	.05178	.05886	.06706	.07253	.07973
21	70.0	.03205	.03677	.04007	.04492	.05054	.05463	.06043
22	72.5	.02465	.02713	.02889	.03150	.03455	.03728	.04166
23	75.0	.01823	.01964	.02065	.02217	.02402	.02573	.02860
24	77.5	.01218	.01287	.01338	.01415	.01509	.01607	.01789
25	80.0	.00781	.00813	.00837	.00873	.00918	.00971	.01080

TABLE A.I.6.   SOUTH MODEL VALUES FOR FEMALE PROBABILITIES OF DYING, $q(x)$

Level	e_0	$q(1)$	$q(2)$	$q(3)$	$q(5)$	$q(10)$	$q(15)$	$q(20)$
1	20.0	.30700	.44469	.50808	.56057	.60018	.61944	.64448
2	22.5	.28449	.41367	.47315	.52240	.56140	.58060	.60571
3	25.0	.26415	.38496	.44059	.48664	.52462	.54354	.56844
4	27.5	.24563	.35824	.41008	.45301	.48966	.50812	.53256
5	30.0	.22865	.33324	.38140	.42128	.45635	.47421	.49799
6	32.5	.21298	.30978	.35435	.39125	.42456	.44169	.46464
7	35.0	.19847	.28769	.32876	.36278	.39415	.41407	.43246
8	37.5	.18496	.26682	.30450	.33571	.36504	.38046	.40137
9	40.0	.17234	.24705	.28145	.30993	.33712	.35158	.37132
10	42.5	.16065	.22823	.25935	.28511	.30969	.32315	.34185
11	45.0	.15044	.21077	.23855	.26155	.28367	.29599	.31318
12	47.5	.14047	.19397	.21860	.23900	.25873	.26990	.28556
13	50.0	.13075	.17781	.19948	.21741	.23481	.24483	.25896
14	52.5	.12130	.16226	.18112	.19674	.21185	.22073	.23334
15	55.0	.11214	.14732	.16351	.17692	.18982	.19756	.20866
16	57.5	.10327	.13295	.14661	.15793	.16865	.17529	.18489
17	60.0	.09471	.11899	.13025	.13971	.14832	.15385	.16198
18	62.5	.08639	.10546	.11411	.12209	.12869	.13312	.13978
19	65.0	.07715	.09199	.09906	.10526	.11051	.11408	.11924
20	67.5	.06801	.07930	.08475	.08964	.09359	.09637	.10038
21	70.0	.05890	.06717	.07122	.07493	.07778	.07985	.08285
22	72.5	.04987	.05564	.05849	.06117	.06311	.06458	.06672
23	75.0	.04096	.04472	.04661	.04842	.04965	.05063	.05205
24	77.5	.03226	.03450	.03564	.03676	.03746	.03805	.03891
25	80.0	.02486	.02614	.02679	.02745	.02783	.02817	.02867

TABLE A.I.7.   EAST MODEL VALUES FOR FEMALE PROBABILITIES OF DYING, $q(x)$

Level	e_0	$q(1)$	$q(2)$	$q(3)$	$q(5)$	$q(10)$	$q(15)$	$q(20)$
1	20.0	.42785	.50168	.53306	.56794	.59930	.61558	.63645
2	22.5	.39330	.46469	.49504	.52877	.56000	.57636	.59744
3	25.0	.36180	.43029	.45941	.49177	.52252	.53877	.55981
4	27.5	.33288	.39814	.42588	.45671	.48671	.50269	.52350
5	30.0	.30618	.36796	.39422	.42341	.45243	.46803	.48843
6	32.5	.28141	.33955	.36426	.39172	.41958	.43468	.45452
7	35.0	.25833	.31270	.33582	.36151	.38806	.40256	.42173
8	37.5	.23674	.28728	.30876	.33264	.35776	.37159	.38998
9	40.0	.21648	.26315	.28298	.30503	.32861	.34172	.35923
10	42.5	.19742	.24019	.25837	.27858	.30054	.31287	.32943
11	45.0	.17960	.21787	.23414	.25223	.27232	.28388	.29964
12	47.5	.16300	.19683	.21121	.22720	.24536	.25599	.27058
13	50.0	.14703	.17668	.18929	.20330	.21956	.22923	.24262
14	52.5	.13169	.15741	.16834	.18048	.19487	.20357	.21573
15	55.0	.11698	.13897	.14832	.15871	.17126	.17899	.18990
16	57.5	.10290	.12135	.12920	.13792	.14867	.15543	.16509
17	60.0	.08942	.10431	.11074	.11806	.12705	.13284	.14124
18	62.5	.07657	.08809	.09316	.09908	.10635	.11119	.11834
19	65.0	.06433	.07270	.07646	.08095	.08653	.09043	.09633
20	67.5	.05268	.05811	.06058	.06362	.06754	.07051	.07519
21	70.0	.04093	.04450	.04616	.04824	.05101	.05316	.05651
22	72.5	.03063	.03284	.03389	.03522	.03704	.03852	.04090
23	75.0	.02144	.02266	.02325	.02401	.02508	.02602	.02757
24	77.5	.01360	.01418	.01446	.01483	.01538	.01590	.01678
25	80.0	.00755	.00777	.00788	.00802	.00825	.00849	.00892

TABLE A.I.8.   WEST MODEL VALUES FOR FEMALE PROBABILITIES OF DYING, $q(x)$

Level	e_0	$q(1)$	$q(2)$	$q(3)$	$q(5)$	$q(10)$	$q(15)$	$q(20)$
1	20.0	.36517	.45000	.48801	.53117	.56544	.59028	.62507
2	22.5	.33362	.41443	.45064	.49176	.52555	.55022	.58051
3	25.0	.30519	.38171	.41601	.45494	.48794	.51217	.54214
4	27.5	.27936	.35144	.38375	.42042	.45237	.47596	.50535
5	30.0	.25573	.32329	.35357	.38795	.41865	.44144	.47002
6	32.5	.23398	.29700	.32524	.35730	.38661	.40847	.43606
7	35.0	.21386	.27235	.29885	.32831	.35611	.37693	.40339
8	37.5	.19518	.24916	.27335	.30082	.32702	.34671	.37192
9	40.0	.17774	.22729	.24949	.27470	.29922	.31773	.34158
10	42.5	.16143	.20660	.22685	.24983	.27263	.28989	.31231
11	45.0	.14612	.18700	.20532	.22611	.24715	.26313	.28404
12	47.5	.13171	.16837	.18481	.20346	.22271	.23737	.25673
13	50.0	.11831	.15061	.16508	.18152	.19900	.21229	.23010
14	52.5	.10548	.13280	.14504	.15894	.17441	.18613	.20251
15	55.0	.09339	.11636	.12676	.13873	.15227	.16260	.17716
16	57.5	.08177	.10064	.10934	.11959	.13126	.14020	.15297
17	60.0	.07066	.08581	.09291	.10146	.11132	.11890	.12990
18	62.5	.06004	.07180	.07740	.08429	.09238	.09864	.10789
19	65.0	.04994	.05857	.06276	.06799	.07439	.07935	.08689
20	67.5	.04034	.04608	.04891	.05251	.05725	.06094	.06683
21	70.0	.03093	.03441	.03615	.03840	.04165	.04426	.04842
22	72.5	.02262	.02740	.02575	.02714	.02928	.03102	.03386
23	75.0	.01516	.01623	.01679	.01752	.01877	.01981	.02154
24	77.5	.00894	.00939	.00963	.00994	.01055	.01107	.01197
25	80.0	.00445	.00460	.00467	.00478	.00501	.00522	.00560

TABLE A.I.9.   NORTH MODEL VALUES FOR PROBABILITIES OF DYING, $q(x)$, BOTH SEXES COMBINED[a]

Level	e_0	$q(1)$	$q(2)$	$q(3)$	$q(5)$	$q(10)$	$q(15)$	$q(20)$
1	18.8	.34608	.42815	.47836	.54455	.60282	.62896	.65402
2	21.2	.31620	.39420	.44191	.50481	.56241	.58864	.61407
3	23.6	.28938	.36313	.40825	.46772	.52408	.55011	.57561
4	26.1	.26509	.33451	.37698	.43297	.48765	.51323	.53856
5	28.6	.24292	.30800	.34782	.40030	.45296	.47790	.50284
6	31.0	.22256	.28333	.32050	.36949	.41987	.44400	.46841
7	33.5	.20377	.26026	.29482	.34037	.38826	.41144	.43517
8	36.0	.18635	.23863	.27062	.31277	.35802	.38016	.40308
9	38.4	.17012	.21829	.24775	.28658	.32904	.35005	.37207
10	40.9	.15496	.19909	.22609	.26166	.30127	.32106	.34209
11	43.4	.14076	.18095	.20553	.23793	.27459	.29313	.31311
12	45.9	.12744	.16379	.18602	.21533	.24902	.26625	.28513
13	48.3	.11503	.14701	.16657	.19235	.22271	.23862	.25654
14	50.8	.10386	.13158	.14861	.17113	.19815	.21264	.22941
15	53.2	.09300	.11670	.13139	.15096	.17474	.18779	.20332
16	55.7	.08249	.10215	.11473	.13182	.15248	.16407	.17831
17	58.1	.07235	.08837	.09899	.11367	.13131	.14147	.15436
18	60.6	.06262	.07540	.08414	.09645	.11120	.11991	.13145
19	63.1	.05331	.06317	.07015	.08012	.09208	.09938	.10953
20	65.7	.04445	.05167	.05696	.06462	.07388	.07980	.08858
21	68.2	.03602	.04086	.04451	.04989	.05653	.06110	.06851
22	70.7	.02806	.03067	.03271	.03575	.03985	.04309	.04912
23	73.3	.02094	.02247	.02369	.02555	.02820	.03041	.03476
24	75.9	.01417	.01493	.01557	.01655	.01804	.01939	.02242
25	78.6	.00922	.00958	.00963	.01037	.01115	.01195	.01399

[a] With sex ratio at birth of 1.05.

Level	e_0	q(1)	q(2)	q(3)	q(5)	q(10)	q(15)	q(20)
1	19.9	.32162	.45276	.51319	.56335	.60047	.61768	.64117
2	22.4	.29818	.42161	.47850	.52570	.56231	.57949	.60305
3	24.8	.27701	.39279	.44614	.49042	.52613	.54309	.56648
4	27.2	.25772	.36595	.41583	.45723	.49175	.50835	.53133
5	29.6	.24004	.34087	.38733	.42589	.45901	.47512	.49752
6	32.0	.22373	.31731	.36045	.39624	.42777	.44328	.46495
7	34.4	.20862	.29514	.33501	.36811	.39790	.41274	.43356
8	36.8	.19455	.27420	.31090	.34136	.36932	.38341	.40327
9	39.2	.18141	.25436	.28798	.31588	.34191	.35520	.37402
10	41.5	.16929	.23589	.26658	.29205	.31575	.32819	.34606
11	43.9	.15862	.21822	.24569	.26849	.28999	.30150	.31809
12	46.3	.14821	.21022	.22564	.24592	.26525	.27583	.29110
13	48.7	.13806	.18485	.20640	.22430	.24149	.25112	.26506
14	51.0	.12819	.16908	.18793	.20358	.21868	.22734	.23993
15	53.4	.11861	.15393	.17020	.18371	.19677	.20446	.21571
16	55.8	.10934	.13935	.15318	.16466	.17570	.18246	.19235
17	58.1	.10040	.12527	.13678	.14639	.15547	.16127	.16983
18	60.0	.09170	.11154	.12082	.12871	.13589	.14073	.14795
19	63.1	.08178	.09667	.10382	.11011	.11578	.11978	.12559
20	65.6	.07215	.08342	.08898	.09401	.09836	.10158	.10626
21	68.0	.06256	.07077	.07492	.07880	.08201	.08452	.08815
22	70.5	.05304	.05873	.06168	.06451	.06676	.06864	.07135
23	73.0	.04363	.04732	.04929	.05123	.05270	.05403	.05593
24	75.5	.03442	.03662	.03781	.03902	.03990	.04077	.04200
25	78.0	.02658	.02783	.02852	.02924	.02974	.03028	.03105

[a] With sex ratio at birth of 1.05.

Level	e_0	q(1)	q(2)	q(3)	q(5)	q(10)	q(15)	q(20)
1	18.7	.46740	.53686	.56608	.59837	.62691	.64059	.65908
2	21.2	.42976	.49761	.52614	.55768	.58639	.60028	.61918
3	23.7	.39546	.46107	.48867	.51917	.54768	.56161	.58067
4	26.2	.36396	.42691	.45337	.48263	.51065	.52446	.54349
5	28.7	.33488	.39482	.42002	.44787	.47515	.48874	.50757
6	31.2	.30791	.36459	.38842	.41476	.44110	.45435	.47282
7	33.6	.28277	.33602	.35841	.38315	.40839	.42121	.43921
8	36.1	.25925	.30895	.32984	.35293	.37692	.38924	.40667
9	38.6	.23719	.28324	.30260	.32400	.34663	.35839	.37514
10	41.0	.21643	.25878	.27658	.29626	.31744	.32859	.34460
11	43.5	.19701	.23499	.25096	.26861	.28806	.29863	.31400
12	45.9	.17907	.21282	.22700	.24267	.26042	.27029	.28478
13	48.3	.16179	.19150	.20399	.21779	.23384	.24295	.25651
14	50.7	.14515	.17103	.18191	.19393	.20827	.21661	.22918
15	53.1	.12917	.15140	.16075	.17107	.18371	.19126	.20279
16	55.6	.11384	.13259	.14047	.14918	.16013	.16687	.17733
17	58.0	.09915	.11447	.12095	.12820	.13748	.14340	.15277
18	60.4	.08513	.09705	.10221	.10811	.11573	.12084	.12911
19	62.8	.07176	.08040	.08428	.08888	.09487	.09916	.10632
20	65.2	.05902	.06465	.06726	.07047	.07485	.07833	.08437
21	67.6	.04631	.05005	.05186	.05415	.05741	.06012	.06490
22	70.0	.03488	.03720	.03836	.03987	.04210	.04411	.04780
23	72.5	.02460	.02589	.02656	.02745	.02883	.03023	.03291
24	75.0	.01576	.01638	.01671	.01715	.01792	.01878	.02056
25	77.6	.00886	.00910	.00923	.00941	.00976	.01024	.01129

[a] With sex ratio at birth of 1.05.

TABLE A.I.12. WEST MODEL VALUES FOR PROBABILITIES OF DYING, $q(x)$, BOTH SEXES COMBINED[a]

Level	e_0	$q(1)$	$q(2)$	$q(3)$	$q(5)$	$q(10)$	$q(15)$	$q(20)$
1	19.0	.39278	.47403	.51004	.55103	.58262	.60468	.63218
2	21.4	.35913	.43699	.47149	.51077	.54211	.56415	.59182
3	23.9	.32882	.40291	.43575	.47312	.50388	.52565	.55318
4	26.4	.30128	.37136	.40242	.43777	.46771	.48900	.51613
5	28.8	.27608	.34202	.37123	.40449	.43339	.45406	.48057
6	31.3	.25289	.31459	.34193	.37306	.40077	.42068	.44640
7	33.7	.23143	.28888	.31433	.34330	.36969	.38875	.41354
8	36.2	.21151	.26469	.28825	.31507	.34005	.35815	.38189
9	38.6	.19292	.24187	.26354	.28823	.31171	.32881	.35139
10	41.1	.17553	.22027	.24010	.26267	.28459	.30062	.32198
11	43.5	.15920	.19980	.21780	.23827	.25861	.27353	.29358
12	46.0	.14383	.18036	.19654	.21496	.23368	.24744	.26614
13	48.5	.12912	.16099	.17511	.19119	.20814	.22061	.23796
14	51.0	.11524	.14247	.15453	.16826	.18342	.19460	.21061
15	53.4	.10259	.12579	.13611	.14795	.16141	.17142	.18593
16	55.8	.09037	.10972	.11843	.12854	.14033	.14914	.16214
17	58.2	.07862	.09415	.10138	.11001	.12015	.12778	.13924
18	60.6	.06734	.07941	.08521	.09233	.10083	.10729	.11721
19	63.1	.05656	.06547	.06989	.07545	.08236	.08765	.09604
20	65.5	.04628	.05229	.05537	.05934	.06469	.06883	.07571
21	68.0	.03604	.03979	.04178	.04440	.04830	.05143	.05675
22	70.5	.02678	.02908	.03033	.03202	.03475	.03698	.04093
23	73.1	.01838	.01960	.02030	.02124	.02297	.02442	.02711
24	75.7	.01118	.01173	.01204	.01248	.01342	.01425	.01587
25	78.3	.00581	.00594	.00611	.00627	.00669	.00708	.00793

[a] With sex ratio at birth of 1.05.

67

ANNEX II
United Nations model life table values for probabilities of dying
between birth and exact age x, $q(x)$

TABLES

		Page
A.II.1.	Latin American model values for male probabilities of dying, $q(x)$	68
A.II.2.	Chilean model values for male probabilities of dying, $q(x)$	69
A.II.3.	South Asian model values for male probabilities of dying, $q(x)$	70
A.II.4.	Far Eastern model values for male probabilities of dying, $q(x)$	70
A.II.5.	General model values for male probabilities of dying, $q(x)$	71
A.II.6.	Latin American model values for female probabilities of dying, $q(x)$	72
A.II.7.	Chilean model values for female probabilities of dying, $q(x)$	72
A.II.8.	South Asian model values for female probabilities of dying, $q(x)$	73
A.II.9.	Far Eastern model values for female probabilities of dying, $q(x)$	74
A.II.10.	General model values for female probabilities of dying, $q(x)$	74
A.II.11.	Latin American model values for probabilities of dying, $q(x)$, both sexes combined	75
A.II.12.	Chilean model values for probabilities of dying, $q(x)$, both sexes combined	76
A.II.13.	South Asian model values for probabilities of dying, $q(x)$, both sexes combined	76
A.II.14.	Far Eastern model values for probabilities of dying, $q(x)$, both sexes combined	77
A.II.15.	General model values for probabilities of dying, $q(x)$, both sexes combined	78

TABLE A.II.1. LATIN AMERICAN MODEL VALUES FOR MALE PROBABILITIES OF DYING, $q(x)$

Level	e_0	$q(1)$	$q(2)$	$q(3)$	$q(5)$	$q(10)$	$q(15)$	$q(20)$
1	35	.20429	.26825	.30174	.33663	.36840	.38433	.40543
2	36	.19839	.25985	.29204	.32562	.35637	.37187	.39248
3	37	.19260	.25161	.28251	.31481	.34454	.35961	.37973
4	38	.18690	.24352	.27316	.30420	.33291	.34754	.36716
5	39	.18129	.23556	.26397	.29376	.32147	.33567	.35478
6	40	.17577	.22774	.25494	.28352	.31022	.32399	.34258
7	41	.17033	.22005	.24607	.27345	.29916	.31249	.33057
8	42	.16497	.21249	.23735	.26355	.28829	.30118	.31874
9	43	.15969	.20506	.22878	.25383	.27760	.29006	.30709
10	44	.15448	.19775	.22036	.24428	.26709	.27912	.29561
11	45	.14934	.19056	.21209	.23490	.25676	.26836	.28432
12	46	.14427	.18348	.20395	.22568	.24661	.25778	.27321
13	47	.13927	.17652	.19596	.21663	.23664	.24737	.26227
14	48	.13433	.16967	.18810	.20774	.22684	.23715	.25151
15	49	.12945	.16293	.18039	.19901	.21722	.22711	.24093
16	50	.12464	.15630	.17280	.19043	.20777	.21724	.23053
17	51	.11988	.14978	.16535	.18202	.19850	.20755	.22031
18	52	.11518	.14337	.15804	.17377	.18940	.19804	.21027
19	53	.11055	.13706	.15086	.16568	.18048	.18871	.20041
20	54	.10597	.13086	.14381	.15774	.17173	.17956	.19073
21	55	.10144	.12476	.13689	.14996	.16316	.17059	.18124
22	56	.09697	.11877	.13010	.14234	.15476	.16180	.17194
23	57	.09256	.11289	.12345	.13487	.14653	.15320	.16282
24	58	.08821	.10711	.11692	.12757	.13849	.14478	.15389
25	59	.08391	.10144	.11054	.12042	.13063	.13654	.14516
26	60	.07967	.09588	.10429	.11345	.12295	.12850	.13662
27	61	.07550	.09043	.09818	.10663	.11546	.12066	.12829
28	62	.07138	.08510	.09221	.09999	.10816	.11301	.12017
29	63	.06733	.07988	.08639	.09352	.10106	.10557	.11255
30	64	.06335	.07478	.08071	.08722	.09415	.09833	.10455
31	65	.05943	.06980	.07518	.08110	.08744	.09130	.09708
32	66	.05559	.06495	.06980	.07516	.08094	.08448	.08982
33	67	.05181	.06022	.06458	.06940	.07464	.07789	.08280
34	68	.04812	.05563	.05952	.06384	.06857	.07152	.07603
35	69	.04452	.05117	.05463	.05848	.06271	.06539	.06950

TABLE A.II.1. (*continued*)

Level	e_0	q(1)	q(2)	q(3)	q(5)	q(10)	q(15)	q(20)
36	70	.04100	.04686	.04991	.05331	.05709	.05950	.06322
37	71	.03758	.04270	.04537	.04836	.05170	.05386	.05721
38	72	.03426	.03870	.04101	.04362	.04655	.04847	.05147
39	73	.03105	.03486	.03685	.03910	.04165	.04335	.04601
40	74	.02795	.03120	.03289	.03481	.03702	.03849	.04084
41	75	.02499	.02771	.02914	.03077	.03265	.03393	.03598

TABLE A.II.2. CHILEAN MODEL VALUES FOR MALE PROBABILITIES OF DYING, $q(x)$

Level	e_0	q(1)	q(2)	q(3)	q(5)	q(10)	q(15)	q(20)
1	35	.23869	.27532	.29384	.31352	.33309	.34705	.36922
2	36	.23135	.26628	.28395	.30277	.32155	.33505	.35656
3	37	.22413	.25741	.27426	.29223	.31025	.32328	.34413
4	38	.21702	.24870	.26475	.28190	.29917	.31173	.33193
5	39	.21003	.24015	.25542	.27178	.28832	.30042	.31996
6	40	.20314	.23176	.24628	.26185	.27767	.28931	.30820
7	41	.19636	.22352	.23730	.25212	.26724	.27843	.29666
8	42	.18968	.21542	.22850	.24258	.25701	.26775	.28533
9	43	.18310	.20748	.21986	.23323	.24698	.25729	.27421
10	44	.17661	.19967	.21139	.22406	.23715	.24702	.26331
11	45	.17022	.19200	.20307	.21507	.22752	.23696	.25261
12	46	.16393	.18446	.19491	.20625	.21807	.22710	.24211
13	47	.15772	.17706	.18691	.19761	.20882	.21744	.23182
14	48	.15161	.16979	.17906	.18915	.19976	.20797	.22173
15	49	.14558	.16265	.17135	.18085	.19089	.19869	.21185
16	50	.13964	.15564	.16380	.17273	.18219	.18961	.20216
17	51	.13379	.14875	.15640	.16477	.17369	.18072	.19267
18	52	.12803	.14200	.14914	.15697	.16536	.17202	.18338
19	53	.12236	.13537	.14202	.14934	.15722	.16351	.17429
20	54	.11677	.12887	.13506	.14188	.14925	.15519	.16541
21	55	.11128	.12249	.12824	.13458	.14148	.14706	.15672
22	56	.10587	.11624	.12156	.12745	.13388	.13912	.14823
23	57	.10055	.11012	.11503	.12048	.12646	.13137	.13995
24	58	.09532	.10412	.10865	.11368	.11922	.12381	.13186
25	59	.09019	.09826	.10241	.10704	.11216	.11644	.12398
26	60	.08515	.09252	.09632	.10056	.10529	.10927	.11631
27	61	.08021	.08692	.09039	.09426	.09861	.10229	.10885
28	62	.07537	.08146	.08461	.08814	.09211	.09552	.10161
29	63	.07063	.07614	.07898	.08219	.08581	.08895	.09458
30	64	.06601	.07096	.07352	.07642	.07971	.08258	.08778
31	65	.06149	.06592	.06822	.07083	.07381	.07643	.08120
32	66	.05710	.06104	.06309	.06542	.06811	.07049	.07485
33	67	.05282	.05632	.05814	.06021	.06261	.06477	.06874
34	68	.04868	.05175	.05335	.05519	.05733	.05927	.06287
35	69	.04466	.04735	.04875	.05037	.05226	.05400	.05724
36	70	.04079	.04312	.04434	.04575	.04741	.04896	.05186
37	71	.03706	.03906	.04012	.04134	.04279	.04416	.04674
38	72	.03348	.03519	.03609	.03714	.03840	.03960	.04189
39	73	.03006	.03151	.03227	.03317	.03425	.03529	.03729
40	74	.02681	.02802	.02867	.02942	.03034	.03124	.03298
41	75	.02374	.02474	.02527	.02590	.02667	.02744	.02895

TABLE A.II.3. SOUTH ASIAN MODEL VALUES FOR MALE PROBABILITIES OF DYING, $q(x)$

Level	e_0	q(1)	q(2)	q(3)	q(5)	q(10)	q(15)	q(20)
1	35	.22680	.30531	.34498	.38328	.41247	.42365	.43606
2	36	.22045	.29613	.33437	.37132	.39965	.41055	.42271
3	37	.21419	.28709	.32390	.35952	.38699	.39761	.40950
4	38	.20803	.27818	.31357	.34788	.37448	.38482	.39643
5	39	.20194	.26939	.30339	.33640	.36213	.37219	.38352
6	40	.19594	.26072	.29335	.32507	.34993	.35970	.37075
7	41	.19002	.25217	.28344	.31389	.33789	.34737	.35813
8	42	.18416	.24373	.27367	.30286	.32600	.33519	.34566
9	43	.17838	.23540	.26404	.29199	.31427	.32317	.33333
10	44	.17267	.22719	.25454	.28126	.30269	.31130	.32116
11	45	.16702	.21908	.24516	.27069	.29127	.29958	.30914
12	46	.16143	.21108	.23592	.26026	.28000	.28802	.29727
13	47	.15591	.20318	.22681	.24999	.26889	.27662	.28556
14	48	.15044	.19539	.21782	.23986	.25794	.26537	.27400
15	49	.14503	.18771	.20897	.22989	.24715	.25429	.26261
16	50	.13968	.18013	.20025	.22007	.23653	.24337	.25137
17	51	.13439	.17265	.19165	.21041	.22607	.23261	.24030
18	52	.12914	.16527	.18319	.20089	.21577	.22203	.22940
19	53	.12396	.15800	.17486	.19154	.20564	.21161	.21867
20	54	.11882	.15083	.16666	.18234	.19568	.20137	.20811
21	55	.11375	.14378	.15860	.17331	.18590	.19130	.19774
22	56	.10872	.13683	.15068	.16444	.17630	.18141	.18754
23	57	.10375	.12998	.14289	.15574	.16687	.17172	.17753
24	58	.09884	.12325	.13525	.14720	.15764	.16221	.16772
25	59	.09398	.11664	.12775	.13884	.14859	.15289	.15809
26	60	.08918	.11014	.12040	.13066	.13974	.14377	.14868
27	61	.08444	.10376	.11320	.12266	.13109	.13486	.13947
28	62	.07977	.09751	.10616	.11485	.12265	.12617	.13048
29	63	.07517	.09139	.09929	.10724	.11442	.11769	.12172
30	64	.07063	.08540	.09258	.09982	.10642	.10944	.11320
31	65	.06617	.07955	.08605	.09262	.09865	.10144	.10491
32	66	.06179	.07386	.07971	.08564	.09112	.09368	.09688
33	67	.05750	.06831	.07355	.07887	.08383	.08617	.08911
34	68	.05329	.06293	.06760	.07234	.07680	.07893	.08162
35	69	.04919	.05772	.06184	.06605	.07004	.07196	.07441
36	70	.04519	.05269	.05631	.06001	.06355	.06528	.06749
37	71	.04131	.04785	.05100	.05423	.05736	.05889	.06088
38	72	.03755	.04320	.04592	.04873	.05146	.05282	.05459
39	73	.03393	.03876	.04109	.04350	.04587	.04706	.04863
40	74	.03045	.03454	.03652	.03856	.04060	.04164	.04301
41	75	.02713	.03056	.03221	.03393	.03566	.03656	.03775

TABLE A.II.4. FAR EASTERN MODEL VALUES FOR MALE PROBABILITIES OF DYING, $q(x)$

Level	e_0	q(1)	q(2)	q(3)	q(5)	q(10)	q(15)	q(20)
1	35	.16455	.20614	.22919	.25567	.28513	.30681	.33721
2	36	.15873	.19819	.22008	.24528	.27346	.29434	.32377
3	37	.15304	.19044	.21120	.23515	.26208	.28217	.31063
4	38	.14746	.18287	.20254	.22528	.25098	.27028	.29777
5	39	.14200	.17548	.19409	.21566	.24015	.25868	.28519
6	40	.13664	.16827	.18586	.20628	.22960	.24735	.27289
7	41	.13139	.16122	.17782	.19714	.21931	.23630	.26086
8	42	.12624	.15434	.16999	.18824	.20928	.22552	.24911
9	43	.12119	.14762	.16234	.17955	.19950	.21500	.23763
10	44	.11623	.14105	.15489	.17110	.18997	.20475	.22642
11	45	.11137	.13464	.14762	.16286	.18070	.19475	.21547
12	46	.10660	.12838	.14053	.15484	.17166	.18502	.20479
13	47	.10192	.12226	.13362	.14702	.16287	.17553	.19438
14	48	.09733	.11629	.12689	.13942	.15431	.16630	.18422
15	49	.09282	.11046	.12033	.13202	.14598	.15731	.17433
16	50	.08840	.10477	.11394	.12482	.13789	.14857	.16469
17	51	.08470	.09923	.10772	.11783	.13003	.14008	.15532
18	52	.07982	.09382	.10167	.11104	.12240	.13183	.14622
19	53	.07566	.08855	.09579	.10445	.11500	.12383	.13737
20	54	.07159	.08342	.09007	.09805	.10784	.11608	.12880
21	55	.06760	.07843	.08453	.09186	.10090	.10858	.12048

TABLE A.II.4.   (*continued*)

Level	e_0	q(1)	q(2)	q(3)	q(5)	q(10)	q(15)	q(20)
22	56	.06370	.07358	.07915	.08586	.09419	.10132	.11244
23	57	.05989	.06887	.07394	.08007	.08771	.09431	.10466
24	58	.05617	.06430	.06890	.07447	.08146	.08755	.09715
25	59	.05254	.05988	.06403	.06907	.07544	.08104	.08992
26	60	.04901	.05559	.05932	.06388	.06965	.07479	.08296
27	61	.04557	.05145	.05479	.05888	.06410	.06878	.07629
28	62	.04224	.04746	.05044	.05409	.05878	.06303	.06989
29	63	.03901	.04363	.04626	.04950	.05369	.05754	.06378
30	64	.03588	.03994	.04226	.04512	.04885	.05231	.05796
31	65	.03287	.03641	.03844	.04095	.04425	.04734	.05242
32	66	.02998	.03304	.03480	.03699	.03989	.04264	.04719
33	67	.02720	.02983	.03135	.03325	.03578	.03820	.04225
34	68	.02455	.02680	.02809	.02973	.03191	.03404	.03762
35	69	.02203	.02393	.02503	.02642	.02829	.03015	.03328
36	70	.01965	.02123	.02216	.02333	.02493	.02652	.02926
37	71	.01740	.01872	.01948	.02046	.02181	.02318	.02553
38	72	.01530	.01638	.01701	.01782	.01894	.02010	.02212
39	73	.01335	.01422	.01473	.01539	.01632	.01729	.01900
40	74	.01155	.01224	.01265	.01319	.01394	.01475	.01618
41	75	.00990	.01045	.01077	.01120	.01180	.01247	.01365

TABLE A.II.5.   GENERAL MODEL VALUES FOR MALE PROBABILITIES OF DYING, $q(x)$

Level	e_0	q(1)	q(2)	q(3)	q(5)	q(10)	q(15)	q(20)
1	35	.20001	.25388	.28242	.31326	.34387	.36121	.38482
2	36	.19387	.24542	.27275	.30233	.33184	.34866	.37165
3	37	.18785	.23713	.26326	.29161	.32003	.33633	.35870
4	38	.18192	.22900	.25396	.28110	.30845	.32422	.34597
5	39	.17609	.22101	.24485	.27080	.29708	.31233	.33345
6	40	.17036	.21318	.23590	.26069	.28592	.30065	.32114
7	41	.16471	.20549	.22713	.25078	.27498	.28919	.30903
8	42	.15915	.19793	.21852	.24107	.26424	.27793	.29713
9	43	.15368	.19052	.21008	.23154	.25371	.26688	.28544
10	44	.14828	.18323	.20179	.22220	.24337	.25604	.27395
11	45	.14297	.17608	.19366	.21304	.23324	.24540	.26266
12	46	.13773	.16905	.18569	.20406	.22331	.23496	.25157
13	47	.13256	.16215	.17787	.19526	.21357	.22472	.24069
14	48	.12747	.15538	.17020	.18663	.20402	.21469	.23001
15	49	.12244	.14872	.16269	.17819	.19468	.20485	.21954
16	50	.11749	.14219	.15531	.16991	.18552	.19521	.20927
17	51	.11261	.13577	.14809	.16181	.17656	.18578	.19920
18	52	.10779	.12948	.14101	.15388	.16779	.17654	.18934
19	53	.10305	.12330	.13408	.14613	.15921	.16751	.17968
20	54	.09837	.11725	.12729	.13855	.15083	.15867	.17023
21	55	.09376	.11131	.12064	.13113	.14264	.15004	.16100
22	56	.08922	.10549	.11414	.12389	.13465	.14161	.15197
23	57	.08475	.09978	.10779	.11683	.12685	.13338	.14316
24	58	.08035	.09421	.10159	.10994	.11925	.12537	.13456
25	59	.07602	.08875	.09553	.10323	.11185	.11757	.12619
26	60	.07177	.08342	.08963	.09670	.10466	.10998	.11805
27	61	.06759	.07821	.08388	.09035	.09767	.10261	.11014
28	62	.06349	.07314	.07829	.08418	.09090	.09546	.10246
29	63	.05947	.06820	.07286	.07820	.08434	.08854	.09502
30	64	.05554	.06339	.06759	.07242	.07799	.08185	.08782
31	65	.05170	.05873	.06249	.06683	.07187	.07539	.08088
32	66	.04795	.05420	.05756	.06143	.06597	.06917	.07419
33	67	.04430	.04983	.05280	.05625	.06031	.06320	.06777
34	68	.04075	.04561	.04822	.05127	.05488	.05748	.06161
35	69	.03731	.04155	.04383	.04650	.04969	.05202	.05573
36	70	.03399	.03765	.03963	.04196	.04475	.04682	.05014
37	71	.03079	.03393	.03563	.03764	.04007	.04189	.04484
38	72	.02772	.03039	.03184	.03355	.03565	.03724	.03983
39	73	.02478	.02703	.02825	.02970	.03149	.03287	.03514
40	74	.02200	.02386	.02488	.02610	.02761	.02879	.03075
41	75	.01937	.02089	.02173	.02274	.02400	.02501	.02669

Table A.II.6. Latin American model values for female probabilities of dying, $q(x)$

Level	e_0	$q(1)$	$q(2)$	$q(3)$	$q(5)$	$q(10)$	$q(15)$	$q(20)$
1	35	.16750	.24014	.28091	.32422	.36255	.38118	.40680
2	36	.16339	.23350	.27276	.31447	.35150	.36955	.39437
3	37	.15935	.22697	.26475	.30488	.34063	.35810	.38212
4	38	.15537	.22055	.25688	.29546	.32995	.34685	.37007
5	39	.15144	.21424	.24913	.28620	.31944	.33577	.35820
6	40	.14757	.20802	.24152	.27710	.30911	.32487	.34652
7	41	.14375	.20189	.23403	.26815	.29895	.31415	.33501
8	42	.13998	.19585	.22665	.25935	.28895	.30360	.32368
9	43	.13625	.18989	.21939	.25069	.27911	.29321	.31253
10	44	.13256	.18402	.21224	.24217	.26943	.28299	.30155
11	45	.12891	.17823	.20519	.23379	.25991	.27293	.29073
12	46	.12530	.17252	.19825	.22554	.25054	.26303	.28009
13	47	.12172	.16688	.19142	.21742	.24132	.25329	.26962
14	48	.11818	.16132	.18468	.20944	.23226	.24371	.25931
15	49	.11466	.15582	.17804	.20158	.22333	.23428	.24917
16	50	.11118	.15040	.17150	.19385	.21456	.22500	.23919
17	51	.10772	.14504	.16506	.18624	.20593	.21588	.22938
18	52	.10429	.13975	.15871	.17876	.19745	.20691	.21973
19	53	.10089	.13452	.15245	.17139	.18911	.19810	.21025
20	54	.09751	.12936	.14628	.16415	.18091	.18943	.20093
21	55	.09415	.12426	.14020	.15703	.17285	.18091	.19178
22	56	.09081	.11923	.13421	.15003	.16494	.17255	.18280
23	57	.08749	.11426	.12832	.14315	.15717	.16435	.17398
24	58	.08420	.10935	.12252	.13640	.14955	.15630	.16533
25	59	.08093	.10451	.11681	.12976	.14207	.14840	.15686
26	60	.07767	.09973	.11119	.12325	.13474	.14067	.14856
27	61	.07444	.09502	.10566	.11687	.12756	.13310	.14044
28	62	.07123	.09037	.10023	.11061	.12054	.12569	.13250
29	63	.06804	.08579	.09490	.10448	.11367	.11844	.12475
30	64	.06488	.08128	.08967	.09848	.10695	.11137	.11718
31	65	.06174	.07684	.08454	.09261	.10040	.10447	.10980
32	66	.05862	.07248	.07951	.08688	.09400	.09774	.10262
33	67	.05552	.06819	.07459	.08129	.08778	.09120	.09564
34	68	.05246	.06398	.06977	.07584	.08173	.08483	.08886
35	69	.04943	.05986	.06508	.07054	.07586	.07867	.08230
36	70	.04643	.05582	.06050	.06539	.07016	.07270	.07595
37	71	.04347	.05187	.05604	.06040	.06466	.06693	.06983
38	72	.04055	.04803	.05172	.05557	.05935	.06137	.06393
39	73	.03767	.04428	.04753	.05091	.05424	.05602	.05828
40	74	.03485	.04064	.04348	.04643	.04934	.05090	.05286
41	75	.03209	.03713	.03958	.04213	.04465	.04601	.04771

Table A.II.7. Chilean model values for female probabilities of dying, $q(x)$

Level	e_0	$q(1)$	$q(2)$	$q(3)$	$q(5)$	$q(10)$	$q(15)$	$q(20)$
1	35	.21831	.26540	.28914	.31380	.33696	.35412	.38324
2	36	.21287	.25805	.28081	.30445	.32669	.34321	.37126
3	37	.20750	.25083	.27263	.29527	.31662	.33251	.35950
4	38	.20220	.24373	.26459	.28627	.30673	.32201	.34795
5	39	.19697	.23673	.25669	.27742	.29702	.31170	.33660
6	40	.19180	.22985	.24892	.26873	.28749	.30158	.32547
7	41	.18669	.22307	.24128	.26019	.27813	.29164	.31452
8	42	.18163	.21639	.23375	.25180	.26894	.28187	.30377
9	43	.17663	.20980	.22635	.24354	.25990	.27227	.29321
10	44	.17168	.20330	.21906	.23543	.25102	.26285	.28284
11	45	.16677	.19690	.21188	.22744	.24229	.25358	.27264
12	46	.16192	.19057	.20481	.21959	.23371	.24447	.26263
13	47	.15710	.18433	.19784	.21186	.22528	.23552	.25279
14	48	.15233	.17818	.19097	.20426	.21699	.22673	.24313
15	49	.14759	.17210	.18421	.19677	.20883	.21809	.23363
16	50	.14290	.16610	.17754	.18941	.20082	.20959	.22431
17	51	.13824	.16017	.17097	.18216	.19294	.20125	.21516
18	52	.13363	.15432	.16449	.17504	.18520	.19305	.20618
19	53	.12904	.14854	.15810	.16802	.17759	.18500	.19736
20	54	.12449	.14283	.15181	.16112	.17011	.17709	.18871
21	55	.11998	.13720	.14561	.15433	.16276	.16932	.18022

Level	e_0	q(1)	q(2)	q(3)	q(5)	q(10)	q(15)	q(20)
22	56	.11550	.13164	.13950	.14765	.15554	.16170	.17190
23	57	.11106	.12615	.13349	.14109	.14846	.15422	.16375
24	58	.10665	.12073	.12756	.13463	.14150	.14688	.15576
25	59	.10228	.11538	.12173	.12829	.13468	.13969	.14794
26	60	.09795	.11011	.11599	.12206	.12798	.13264	.14029
27	61	.09365	.10490	.11034	.11595	.12142	.12574	.13280
28	62	.08938	.09978	.10478	.10995	.11499	.11898	.12549
29	63	.08517	.09473	.09932	.10406	.10870	.11237	.11835
30	64	.08099	.08976	.09396	.09830	.10254	.10592	.11138
31	65	.07686	.08488	.08871	.09266	.09653	.09961	.10460
32	66	.07278	.08008	.08356	.08714	.09066	.09347	.09799
33	67	.06875	.07537	.07851	.08176	.08494	.08749	.09157
34	68	.06478	.07075	.07358	.07650	.07936	.08167	.08535
35	69	.06086	.06623	.06877	.07138	.07395	.07602	.07931
36	70	.05702	.06181	.06408	.06640	.06869	.07055	.07347
37	71	.05324	.05750	.05951	.06157	.06360	.06525	.06784
38	72	.04954	.05330	.05507	.05688	.05867	.06013	.06241
39	73	.04591	.04922	.05077	.05235	.05392	.05520	.05719
40	74	.04238	.04526	.04661	.04798	.04934	.05046	.05219
41	75	.03895	.04144	.04260	.04378	.04496	.04592	.04741

TABLE A.II.8. SOUTH ASIAN MODEL VALUES FOR FEMALE PROBABILITIES OF DYING, $q(x)$

Level	e_0	q(1)	q(2)	q(3)	q(5)	q(10)	q(15)	q(20)
1	35	.20275	.28410	.32720	.36998	.40323	.41669	.43606
2	36	.19788	.27649	.31804	.35929	.39145	.40450	.42327
3	37	.19307	.26897	.30901	.34874	.37982	.39246	.41064
4	38	.18831	.26155	.30009	.33833	.36834	.38057	.39815
5	39	.18362	.25423	.29129	.32806	.35701	.36883	.38582
6	40	.17897	.24699	.28260	.31792	.34582	.35724	.37363
7	41	.17438	.23985	.27403	.30791	.33477	.34579	.36159
8	42	.16983	.23278	.26555	.29804	.32387	.33449	.34969
9	43	.16532	.22579	.25719	.28829	.31310	.32332	.33794
10	44	.16085	.21888	.24892	.27867	.30247	.31230	.32634
11	45	.15641	.21204	.24075	.26917	.29198	.30142	.31488
12	46	.15202	.20528	.23268	.25980	.28162	.29068	.30357
13	47	.14765	.19859	.22471	.25054	.27140	.28007	.29241
14	48	.14332	.19197	.21684	.24141	.26132	.26961	.28139
15	49	.13901	.18542	.20905	.23240	.25137	.25929	.27052
16	50	.13474	.17893	.20136	.22351	.24156	.24911	.25980
17	51	.13049	.17251	.19377	.21474	.23189	.23908	.24923
18	52	.12626	.16616	.18627	.20609	.22235	.22918	.23882
19	53	.12206	.15987	.17886	.19757	.21296	.21944	.22855
20	54	.11788	.15365	.17155	.18917	.20370	.20984	.21845
21	55	.11372	.14750	.16433	.18089	.19459	.20039	.20851
22	56	.10959	.14141	.15721	.17274	.18563	.19109	.19872
23	57	.10548	.13539	.15018	.16471	.17681	.18194	.18911
24	58	.10138	.12944	.14325	.15681	.16814	.17296	.17966
25	59	.09731	.12356	.13642	.14904	.15961	.16413	.17038
26	60	.09326	.11774	.12969	.14141	.15124	.15545	.16127
27	61	.08923	.11200	.12307	.13391	.14304	.14696	.15235
28	62	.08522	.10634	.11656	.12655	.13500	.13863	.14362
29	63	.08124	.10076	.11016	.11934	.12713	.13049	.13508
30	64	.07729	.09526	.10387	.11228	.11943	.12253	.12674
31	65	.07337	.08985	.09771	.10538	.11192	.11476	.11861
32	66	.06947	.08453	.09167	.09864	.10459	.10718	.11069
33	67	.06562	.07930	.08577	.09206	.09746	.09981	.10298
34	68	.06180	.07418	.08000	.08566	.09053	.09265	.09551
35	69	.05803	.06917	.07437	.07943	.08380	.08572	.08827
36	70	.05430	.06427	.06890	.07340	.07729	.07901	.08128
37	71	.05063	.05949	.06359	.06756	.07101	.07253	.07454
38	72	.04702	.05484	.05844	.06192	.06496	.06630	.06806
39	73	.04348	.05033	.05347	.05650	.05915	.06032	.06186
40	74	.04002	.04597	.04868	.05130	.05359	.05461	.05594
41	75	.03664	.04177	.04409	.04633	.04829	.04918	.05031

TABLE A.II.9.   FAR EASTERN MODEL VALUES FOR FEMALE PROBABILITIES OF DYING, $q(x)$

Level	e_0	$q(1)$	$q(2)$	$q(3)$	$q(5)$	$q(10)$	$q(15)$	$q(20)$
1	35	.14593	.19139	.21636	.24413	.27285	.29366	.33631
2	36	.14183	.18529	.20913	.23563	.26310	.28307	.32403
3	37	.13781	.17934	.20207	.22734	.25361	.27275	.31205
4	38	.13387	.17351	.19517	.21926	.24435	.26268	.30035
5	39	.13000	.16782	.18844	.21138	.23532	.25286	.28892
6	40	.12619	.16224	.18186	.20369	.22651	.24329	.27777
7	41	.12244	.15678	.17543	.19618	.21792	.23394	.26688
8	42	.11875	.15142	.16914	.18885	.20953	.22481	.25624
9	43	.11511	.14617	.16298	.18168	.20134	.21591	.24585
10	44	.11153	.14103	.15696	.17468	.19335	.20721	.23570
11	45	.10800	.13598	.15106	.16784	.18554	.19872	.22579
12	46	.10451	.13103	.14529	.16115	.17791	.19043	.21612
13	47	.10107	.12616	.13963	.15461	.17047	.18233	.20667
14	48	.09767	.12139	.13409	.14821	.16319	.17442	.19745
15	49	.09431	.11669	.12866	.14195	.15607	.16670	.18844
16	50	.09100	.11208	.12333	.13583	.14913	.15915	.17965
17	51	.08772	.10756	.11812	.12984	.14234	.15179	.17108
18	52	.08448	.10311	.11300	.12399	.13572	.14461	.16272
19	53	.08128	.09874	.10800	.11827	.12925	.13760	.15458
20	54	.07811	.09445	.10309	.11268	.12294	.13076	.14664
21	55	.07498	.09024	.09828	.10721	.11678	.12409	.13891
22	56	.07188	.08610	.09358	.10187	.11078	.11759	.13139
23	57	.06882	.08203	.08897	.09665	.10492	.11126	.12407
24	58	.06580	.07804	.08446	.09156	.09921	.10510	.11696
25	59	.06281	.07413	.08004	.08659	.09366	.09911	.11005
26	60	.05985	.07029	.07573	.08175	.08825	.09328	.10335
27	61	.05694	.06653	.07151	.07703	.08299	.08762	.09685
28	62	.05406	.06284	.06740	.07243	.07788	.08212	.09056
29	63	.05122	.05923	.06338	.06796	.07292	.07680	.08448
30	64	.04842	.05571	.05946	.06361	.06812	.07164	.07860
31	65	.04566	.05226	.05565	.05939	.06346	.06665	.07294
32	66	.04295	.04889	.05194	.05530	.05896	.06184	.06749
33	67	.04028	.04561	.04834	.05134	.05462	.05720	.06224
34	68	.03767	.04242	.04485	.04752	.05043	.05274	.05722
35	69	.03511	.03933	.04147	.04383	.04641	.04845	.05241
36	70	.03260	.03632	.03821	.04028	.04255	.04435	.04783
37	71	.03016	.03342	.03506	.03687	.03885	.04043	.04346
38	72	.02779	.03062	.03204	.03361	.03533	.03670	.03932
39	73	.02548	.02792	.02915	.03050	.03197	.03316	.03541
40	74	.02325	.02534	.02639	.02753	.02879	.02981	.03172
41	75	.02110	.02288	.02376	.02473	.02579	.02665	.02826

TABLE A.II.10.   GENERAL MODEL VALUES FOR FEMALE PROBABILITIES OF DYING, $q(x)$

Level	e_0	$q(1)$	$q(2)$	$q(3)$	$q(5)$	$q(10)$	$q(15)$	$q(20)$
1	35	.16449	.22558	.25960	.29698	.33384	.35454	.38628
2	36	.16030	.21905	.25172	.28762	.32313	.34312	.37379
3	37	.15617	.21265	.24399	.27845	.31262	.33192	.36152
4	38	.15210	.20636	.23641	.26945	.30231	.32092	.34946
5	39	.14810	.20018	.22897	.26063	.29220	.31012	.33762
6	40	.14415	.19410	.22166	.25197	.28228	.29953	.32598
7	41	.14025	.18812	.21448	.24348	.27524	.28912	.31454
8	42	.13640	.18224	.20743	.23514	.26297	.27890	.30331
9	43	.13260	.17645	.20050	.22695	.25358	.26886	.29227
10	44	.12884	.17074	.19368	.21890	.24436	.25901	.28142
11	45	.12512	.16513	.18697	.21100	.23531	.24933	.27077
12	46	.12144	.15959	.18038	.20324	.22643	.23983	.26030
13	47	.11780	.15414	.17389	.19562	.21770	.23049	.25002
14	48	.11419	.14876	.16751	.18813	.20913	.22133	.23993
15	49	.11061	.14346	.16123	.18077	.20072	.21233	.23001
16	50	.10707	.13823	.15505	.17354	.19245	.20349	.22028
17	51	.10356	.13308	.14897	.16644	.18435	.19482	.21073
18	52	.10007	.12799	.14299	.15946	.17639	.18632	.20137
19	53	.09661	.12298	.13710	.15261	.16858	.17796	.19217
20	54	.09318	.11803	.13130	.14588	.16091	.16978	.18316
21	55	.08977	.11314	.12560	.13927	.15340	.16175	.17434

Level	e_0	q(1)	q(2)	q(3)	q(5)	q(10)	q(15)	q(20)
22	56	.08639	.10833	.11999	.13278	.14604	.15388	.16569
23	57	.08304	.10359	.11448	.12642	.13882	.14618	.15723
24	58	.07971	.09891	.10906	.12018	.13175	.13864	.14895
25	59	.07640	.09430	.10373	.11407	.12484	.13126	.14086
26	60	.07312	.08976	.09850	.10808	.11807	.12405	.13296
27	61	.06987	.08529	.09337	.10221	.11146	.11701	.12525
28	62	.06664	.08089	.08833	.09647	.10501	.11014	.11774
29	63	.06344	.07656	.08339	.09086	.09871	.10343	.11042
30	64	.06027	.07230	.07855	.08538	.09257	.09691	.10330
31	65	.05713	.06813	.07382	.08004	.08659	.09056	.09638
32	66	.05402	.06403	.06919	.07483	.08078	.08439	.08968
33	67	.05094	.06001	.06467	.06976	.07513	.07841	.08318
34	68	.04790	.05607	.06026	.06483	.06966	.07262	.07690
35	69	.04490	.05223	.05597	.06005	.06437	.06702	.07085
36	70	.04195	.04848	.05180	.05542	.05926	.06163	.06502
37	71	.03905	.04483	.04776	.05095	.05434	.05644	.05943
38	72	.03620	.04128	.04385	.04664	.04962	.05146	.05408
39	73	.03341	.03785	.04008	.04251	.04509	.04670	.04898
40	74	.03069	.03453	.03645	.03854	.04077	.04217	.04412
41	75	.02804	.03133	.03297	.03476	.03666	.03786	.03953

Table A.II.11.   Latin American model values for probabilities of dying, $q(x)$, both sexes combined[a]

Level	e_0	q(1)	q(2)	q(3)	q(5)	q(10)	q(15)	q(20)
1	35	.18634	.25454	.29158	.33058	.36555	.38279	.40610
2	36	.18132	.24700	.28263	.32018	.35399	.37074	.39340
3	37	.17638	.23959	.27385	.30997	.34263	.35887	.38090
4	38	.17152	.23232	.26522	.29993	.33146	.34720	.36858
5	39	.16673	.22516	.25673	.29007	.32048	.33572	.35645
6	40	.16202	.21812	.24839	.28039	.30968	.32442	.34450
7	41	.15737	.21119	.24019	.27086	.29906	.31330	.33274
8	42	.15278	.20437	.23213	.26150	.28861	.30236	.32115
9	43	.14826	.19766	.22420	.25230	.27834	.29160	.30974
10	44	.14379	.19105	.21640	.24325	.26823	.28101	.29851
11	45	.13938	.18455	.20872	.23436	.25830	.27059	.28745
12	46	.13502	.17813	.20117	.22561	.24853	.26034	.27656
13	47	.13071	.17182	.19374	.21702	.23892	.25026	.26585
14	48	.12645	.16559	.18643	.20857	.22948	.24035	.25531
15	49	.12224	.15946	.17924	.20026	.22020	.23060	.24495
16	50	.11807	.15342	.17217	.19210	.21108	.22103	.23475
17	51	.11395	.14747	.16521	.18408	.20212	.21161	.22473
18	52	.10987	.14160	.15836	.17620	.19333	.20237	.21489
19	53	.10584	.13582	.15163	.16847	.18469	.19329	.20521
20	54	.10184	.13013	.14501	.16087	.17621	.18438	.19571
21	55	.09788	.12452	.13850	.15341	.16788	.17563	.18638
22	56	.09397	.11900	.13211	.14609	.15972	.16705	.17723
23	57	.09009	.11356	.12582	.13891	.15172	.15864	.16826
24	58	.08625	.10820	.11965	.13187	.14388	.15040	.15947
25	59	.08246	.10294	.11360	.12498	.13621	.14233	.15087
26	60	.07870	.09776	.10765	.11823	.12870	.13444	.14245
27	61	.07498	.09267	.10183	.11163	.12137	.12673	.13422
28	62	.07131	.08767	.09613	.10517	.11420	.11919	.12618
29	63	.06768	.08276	.09054	.09886	.10721	.11185	.11835
30	64	.06409	.07795	.08508	.09271	.10039	.10469	.11071
31	65	.06055	.07324	.07974	.08671	.09376	.09772	.10328
32	66	.05706	.06862	.07454	.08088	.08731	.09095	.09607
33	67	.05362	.06411	.06946	.07520	.08105	.08438	.08906
34	68	.05024	.05970	.06452	.06969	.07499	.07802	.08229
35	69	.04691	.05541	.05973	.06436	.06912	.07187	.07574
36	70	.04365	.05123	.05508	.05920	.06347	.06594	.06943
37	71	.04045	.04718	.05058	.05423	.05802	.06023	.06336
38	72	.03733	.04325	.04624	.04945	.05279	.05476	.05755
39	73	.03428	.03946	.04206	.04486	.04779	.04953	.05199
40	74	.03132	.03581	.03806	.04048	.04303	.04455	.04671
41	75	.02845	.03230	.03423	.03631	.03850	.03982	.04170

[a] With sex ratio at birth of 1.05.

TABLE A.II.12.   CHILEAN MODEL VALUES FOR PROBABILITIES OF DYING, $q(x)$, BOTH SEXES COMBINED[a]

Level	e_0	$q(1)$	$q(2)$	$q(3)$	$q(5)$	$q(10)$	$q(15)$	$q(20)$
1	35	.22875	.27048	.29155	.31366	.33497	.35050	.37606
2	36	.22233	.26227	.28242	.30359	.32406	.33903	.36373
3	37	.21602	.25420	.27346	.29371	.31336	.32778	.35163
4	38	.20979	.24627	.26467	.28403	.30286	.31675	.33974
5	39	.20366	.23848	.25604	.27453	.29256	.30592	.32808
6	40	.19761	.23083	.24757	.26521	.28246	.29530	.31662
7	41	.19164	.22330	.23924	.25606	.27255	.28487	.30537
8	42	.18575	.21589	.23106	.24708	.26283	.27464	.29433
9	43	.17994	.20861	.22303	.23826	.25328	.26460	.28348
10	44	.17421	.20144	.21513	.22960	.24392	.25474	.27283
11	45	.16854	.19439	.20737	.22110	.23472	.24507	.26238
12	46	.16295	.18744	.19974	.21276	.22570	.23558	.25212
13	47	.15742	.18061	.19224	.20456	.21685	.22626	.24205
14	48	.15196	.17388	.18487	.19652	.20816	.21712	.23217
15	49	.14656	.16726	.17762	.18862	.19964	.20815	.22247
16	50	.14123	.16074	.17050	.18086	.19128	.19936	.21297
17	51	.13597	.15432	.16350	.17325	.18308	.19073	.20364
18	52	.13076	.14801	.15663	.16578	.17504	.18228	.19450
19	53	.12562	.14179	.14987	.15845	.16715	.17399	.18555
20	54	.12054	.13568	.14323	.15126	.15943	.16587	.17677
21	55	.11552	.12967	.13671	.14422	.15186	.15792	.16818
22	56	.11057	.12375	.13031	.13731	.14445	.15014	.15978
23	57	.10568	.11794	.12404	.13053	.13719	.14252	.15156
24	58	.10085	.11222	.11787	.12390	.13009	.13507	.14352
25	59	.09609	.10661	.11183	.11741	.12314	.12778	.13567
26	60	.09139	.10110	.10591	.11105	.11636	.12067	.12801
27	61	.08676	.09569	.10012	.10484	.10973	.11373	.12054
28	62	.08220	.09040	.09445	.09878	.10327	.10696	.11326
29	63	.07772	.08521	.08890	.09286	.09697	.10037	.10617
30	64	.07332	.08013	.08349	.08709	.09085	.09397	.09929
31	65	.06899	.07517	.07822	.08148	.08489	.08774	.09261
32	66	.06475	.07033	.07308	.07602	.07911	.08170	.08614
33	67	.06059	.06561	.06808	.07072	.07350	.07585	.07988
34	68	.05653	.06102	.06322	.06558	.06808	.07020	.07383
35	69	.05257	.05656	.05852	.06062	.06284	.06474	.06801
36	70	.04870	.05224	.05397	.05582	.05779	.05949	.06240
37	71	.04495	.04806	.04958	.05121	.05294	.05444	.05703
38	72	.04131	.04403	.04535	.04677	.04829	.04962	.05190
39	73	.03780	.04015	.04129	.04253	.04384	.04500	.04700
40	74	.03441	.03643	.03742	.03847	.03961	.04062	.04235
41	75	.03116	.03289	.03372	.03462	.03559	.03646	.03795

[a] With sex ratio at birth of 1.05.

TABLE A.II.13.   SOUTH ASIAN MODEL VALUES FOR PROBABILITIES OF DYING, $q(x)$, BOTH SEXES COMBINED[a]

Level	e_0	$q(1)$	$q(2)$	$q(3)$	$q(5)$	$q(10)$	$q(15)$	$q(20)$
1	35	.21507	.29496	.33631	.37679	.40797	.42025	.43606
2	36	.20944	.28655	.32640	.36545	.39565	.40760	.42298
3	37	.20389	.27825	.31663	.35426	.38349	.39510	.41005
4	38	.19841	.27007	.30700	.34322	.37149	.38275	.39727
5	39	.19300	.26199	.29749	.33233	.35963	.37055	.38464
6	40	.18766	.25402	.28811	.32158	.34792	.35850	.37215
7	41	.18239	.24616	.27885	.31098	.33637	.34660	.35982
8	42	.17717	.23839	.26971	.30051	.32496	.33485	.34763
9	43	.17201	.23071	.26070	.29018	.31370	.32324	.33558
10	44	.16690	.22314	.25180	.28000	.30258	.31179	.32369
11	45	.16185	.21565	.24301	.26995	.29161	.30048	.31194
12	46	.15684	.20825	.23434	.26004	.28079	.28932	.30035
13	47	.15188	.20094	.22579	.25026	.27012	.27830	.28890
14	48	.14697	.19372	.21734	.24062	.25959	.26744	.27761
15	49	.14210	.18659	.20901	.23111	.24921	.25673	.26647
16	50	.13727	.17954	.20079	.22175	.23898	.24617	.25548
17	51	.13248	.17258	.19269	.21252	.22891	.23577	.24466
18	52	.12774	.16570	.18469	.20343	.21898	.22552	.23399
19	53	.12303	.15891	.17681	.19448	.20921	.21543	.22349

Level	e_0	q(1)	q(2)	q(3)	q(5)	q(10)	q(15)	q(20)
20	54	.11836	.15221	.16905	.18567	.19959	.20550	.21316
21	55	.11374	.14559	.16140	.17701	.19014	.19573	.20299
22	56	.10914	.13906	.15386	.16849	.18085	.18613	.19300
23	57	.10459	.13262	.14645	.16011	.17172	.17671	.18318
24	58	.10008	.12627	.13915	.15189	.16276	.16745	.17354
25	59	.09560	.12001	.13198	.14382	.15397	.15837	.16409
26	60	.09117	.00385	.12493	.13590	.14535	.14947	.15482
27	61	.08678	.10778	.11801	.12815	.13692	.14076	.14576
28	62	.08243	.10182	.11123	.12056	.12867	.13225	.13689
29	63	.07813	.09596	.10459	.11314	.12062	.12393	.12824
30	64	.07388	.09021	.09809	.10590	.11277	.11583	.11980
31	65	.06968	.08458	.09174	.09885	.10512	.10793	.11159
32	66	.06554	.07906	.08554	.09198	.09769	.10026	.10362
33	67	.06146	.07368	.07951	.08531	.09048	.09282	.09588
34	68	.05744	.06842	.07365	.07884	.08350	.08562	.08840
35	69	.05350	.06330	.06796	.07258	.07675	.07867	.08117
36	70	.04964	.05834	.06245	.06654	.07026	.07197	.07422
37	71	.04586	.05353	.05714	.06073	.06402	.06555	.06754
38	72	.04217	.04888	.05203	.05516	.05804	.05939	.06116
39	73	.03859	.04441	.04713	.04984	.05234	.05353	.05508
40	74	.03512	.04012	.04245	.04478	.04693	.04797	.04932
41	75	.03177	.03603	.03800	.03998	.04182	.04271	.04388

[a] With sex ratio at birth of 1.05.

TABLE A.II.14.   FAR EASTERN MODEL VALUES FOR PROBABILITIES OF DYING, $q(x)$, BOTH SEXES COMBINED[a]

Level	e_0	q(1)	q(2)	q(3)	q(5)	q(10)	q(15)	q(20)
1	35	.15546	.19895	.22294	.25004	.27914	.30040	.33677
2	36	.15049	.19190	.21474	.24057	.26841	.28884	.32390
3	37	.14561	.18503	.20674	.23134	.25795	.27757	.31132
4	38	.14083	.17831	.19895	.22235	.24775	.26657	.29903
5	39	.13614	.17174	.19134	.21357	.23780	.25584	.28701
6	40	.13154	.16533	.18391	.20502	.22809	.24537	.27527
7	41	.12702	.15905	.17666	.19667	.21863	.23515	.26380
8	42	.12259	.15292	.16957	.18853	.20940	.22518	.25259
9	43	.11823	.14691	.16266	.18059	.20040	.21544	.24164
10	44	.11394	.14104	.15590	.17285	.19162	.20595	.23095
11	45	.10973	.13529	.14930	.16529	.18306	.19669	.22051
12	46	.10558	.12967	.14285	.15791	.17471	.18766	.21032
13	47	.10151	.12417	.13656	.15072	.16657	.17885	.20038
14	48	.09750	.11878	.13040	.14371	.15864	.17026	.19067
15	49	.09355	.11350	.12439	.13686	.15090	.16189	.18121
16	50	.08967	.10834	.11852	.13019	.14337	.15373	.17199
17	51	.08585	.10329	.11279	.12369	.13604	.14579	.16301
18	52	.08209	.09835	.10720	.11736	.12890	.13806	.15427
19	53	.07840	.09352	.10174	.11119	.12195	.13055	.14577
20	54	.07477	.08880	.09642	.10519	.11520	.12324	.13750
21	55	.07120	.08419	.09124	.09935	.10865	.11615	.12947
22	56	.06769	.07969	.08619	.09367	.10228	.10926	.12168
23	57	.06424	.07529	.08127	.08816	.09610	.10258	.11413
24	58	.06086	.07101	.07649	.08281	.09012	.09611	.10681
25	59	.05755	.06683	.07184	.07762	.08433	.08985	.09974
26	60	.05430	.06276	.06733	.07259	.07872	.08381	.09291
27	61	.05112	.05881	.06295	.06773	.07331	.07797	.08632
28	62	.04800	.05497	.05871	.06304	.06810	.07234	.07997
29	63	.04496	.05124	.05461	.05851	.06308	.06693	.07388
30	64	.04200	.04763	.05065	.05414	.05825	.06174	.06803
31	65	.03911	.04414	.04683	.04995	.05362	.05676	.06243
32	66	.03630	.04077	.04316	.04593	.04919	.05201	.05709
33	67	.03358	.03753	.03964	.04208	.04497	.04747	.05200
34	68	.03095	.03442	.03627	.03841	.04095	.04316	.04718
35	69	.02841	.03144	.03305	.03491	.03713	.03908	.04262
36	70	.02597	.02859	.02999	.03160	.03352	.03522	.03832
37	71	.02363	.02589	.02708	.02847	.03012	.03159	.03428

Level	e_0	q(1)	q(2)	q(3)	q(5)	q(10)	q(15)	q(20)
38	72	.02139	.02332	.02434	.02552	.02693	.02820	.03051
39	73	.01927	.02090	.02177	.02276	.02395	.02503	.02700
40	74	.01726	.01863	.01935	.02019	.02119	.02210	.02376
41	75	.01537	.01651	.01711	.01780	.01863	.01939	.02078

[a] With sex ratio at birth of 1.05.

TABLE A.II.15.   GENERAL MODEL VALUES FOR PROBABILITIES OF DYING, $q(x)$, BOTH SEXES COMBINED[a]

Level	e_0	q(1)	q(2)	q(3)	q(5)	q(10)	q(15)	q(20)
1	35	.18268	.24007	.27129	.30531	.33898	.35796	.38533
2	36	.17750	.23526	.26249	.29515	.32759	.34596	.37269
3	37	.17239	.22519	.25386	.28519	.31642	.33417	.36007
4	38	.16738	.21795	.24540	.27542	.30545	.32261	.34767
5	39	.16244	.21085	.23710	.26584	.29470	.31125	.33548
6	40	.15757	.20387	.22895	.25644	.28414	.30010	.32350
7	41	.15278	.19701	.22096	.24722	.27379	.28915	.31172
8	42	.14806	.19028	.21311	.23817	.26362	.27840	.30014
9	43	.14340	.18365	.20540	.22930	.25365	.26785	.28877
10	44	.13880	.17714	.19783	.22059	.24386	.25749	.27759
11	45	.13426	.17074	.19040	.21204	.23425	.24732	.26661
12	46	.12978	.16444	.18310	.20366	.22483	.23733	.25583
13	47	.12536	.15824	.17593	.19543	.21558	.22754	.24524
14	48	.12099	.15215	.16889	.18736	.20651	.21793	.23485
15	49	.11667	.14616	.16198	.17945	.19762	.20850	.22465
16	50	.11241	.14026	.15519	.17168	.18890	.19925	.21464
17	51	.10819	.13446	.14852	.16407	.18036	.19019	.20483
18	52	.10403	.12875	.14197	.15661	.17198	.18131	.19521
19	53	.09991	.12314	.13555	.14929	.16378	.17261	.18578
20	54	.09584	.11763	.12924	.14212	.15575	.16409	.17654
21	55	.09182	.11220	.12306	.13510	.14789	.15575	.16750
22	56	.08784	.10687	.11699	.12823	.14020	.14759	.15866
23	57	.08391	.10164	.11105	.12151	.13269	.13962	.15002
24	58	.08004	.09650	.10523	.11494	.12535	.13184	.14158
25	59	.07621	.09146	.09953	.10852	.11819	.12425	.13335
26	60	.07243	.08651	.09396	.10225	.11120	.11684	.12532
27	61	.06870	.08167	.08851	.09614	.10440	.10963	.11751
28	62	.06503	.07692	.08319	.09018	.09778	.10262	.10991
29	63	.06141	.07228	.07800	.08438	.09135	.09581	.10253
30	64	.05785	.06774	.07294	.07874	.08510	.08919	.09537
31	65	.05435	.06331	.06802	.07327	.07905	.08279	.08844
32	66	.05091	.05900	.06323	.06797	.07319	.07660	.08174
33	67	.04754	.05479	.05859	.06284	.06754	.07062	.07529
34	68	.04424	.05071	.05410	.05788	.06209	.06486	.06907
35	69	.04101	.04676	.04975	.05311	.05685	.05934	.06311
36	70	.03787	.04294	.04557	.04852	.05183	.05404	.05740
37	71	.03482	.03925	.04155	.04413	.04703	.04899	.05196
38	72	.03185	.03570	.03770	.03994	.04246	.04418	.04678
39	73	.02899	.03230	.03402	.03595	.03813	.03962	.04189
40	74	.02624	.02906	.03052	.03217	.03403	.03532	.03728
41	75	.02360	.02598	.02722	.02860	.03018	.03128	.03295

[a] With sex ratio at birth of 1.05.

ANNEX III
Relationship between infant mortality, $q(1)$, and child mortality, $_4q_1$, in the Coale-Demeny mortality models

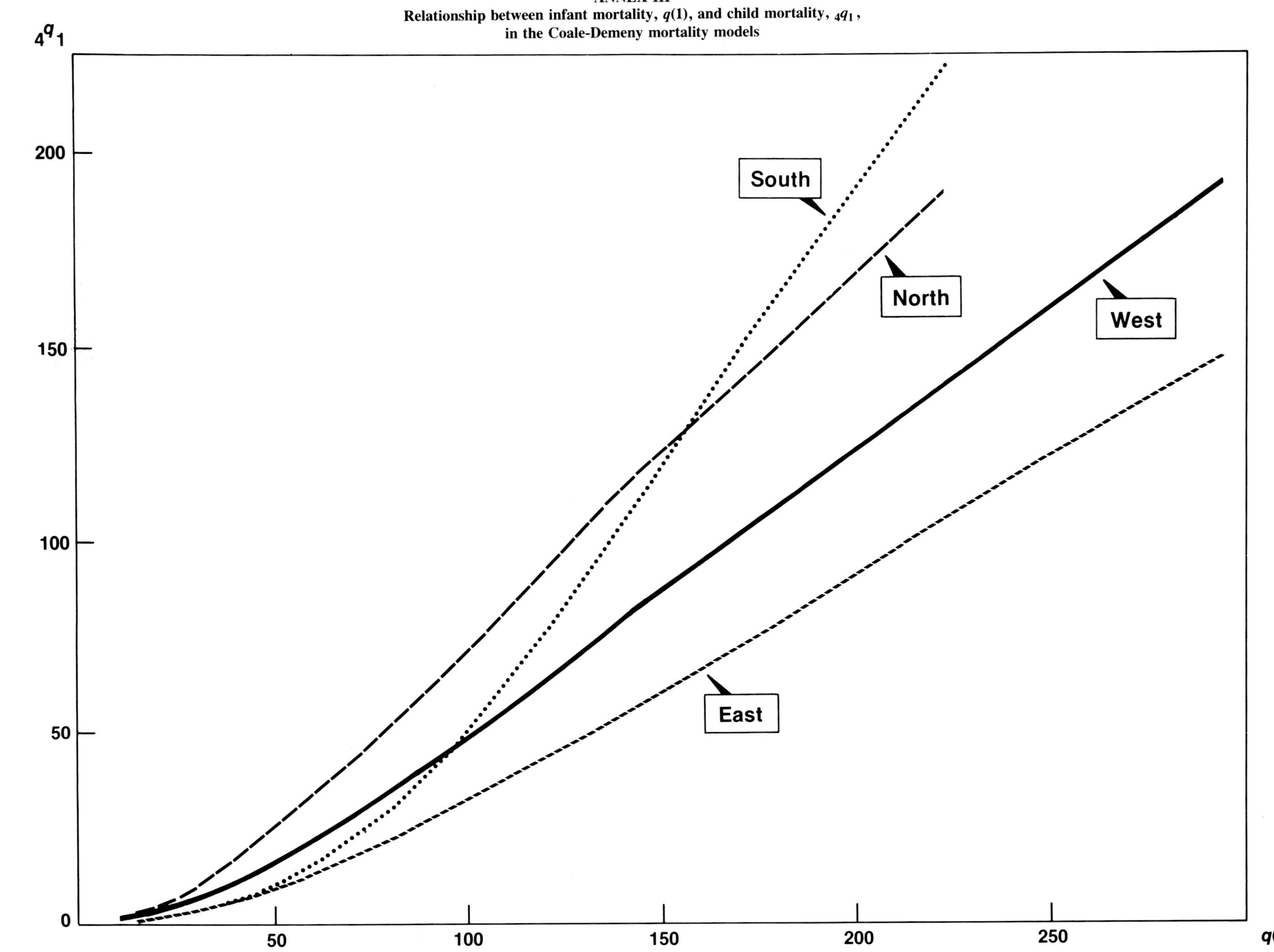

ANNEX IV
Relationship between infant mortality, $q(1)$, and child mortality, $_4q_1$, in the United Nations mortality models

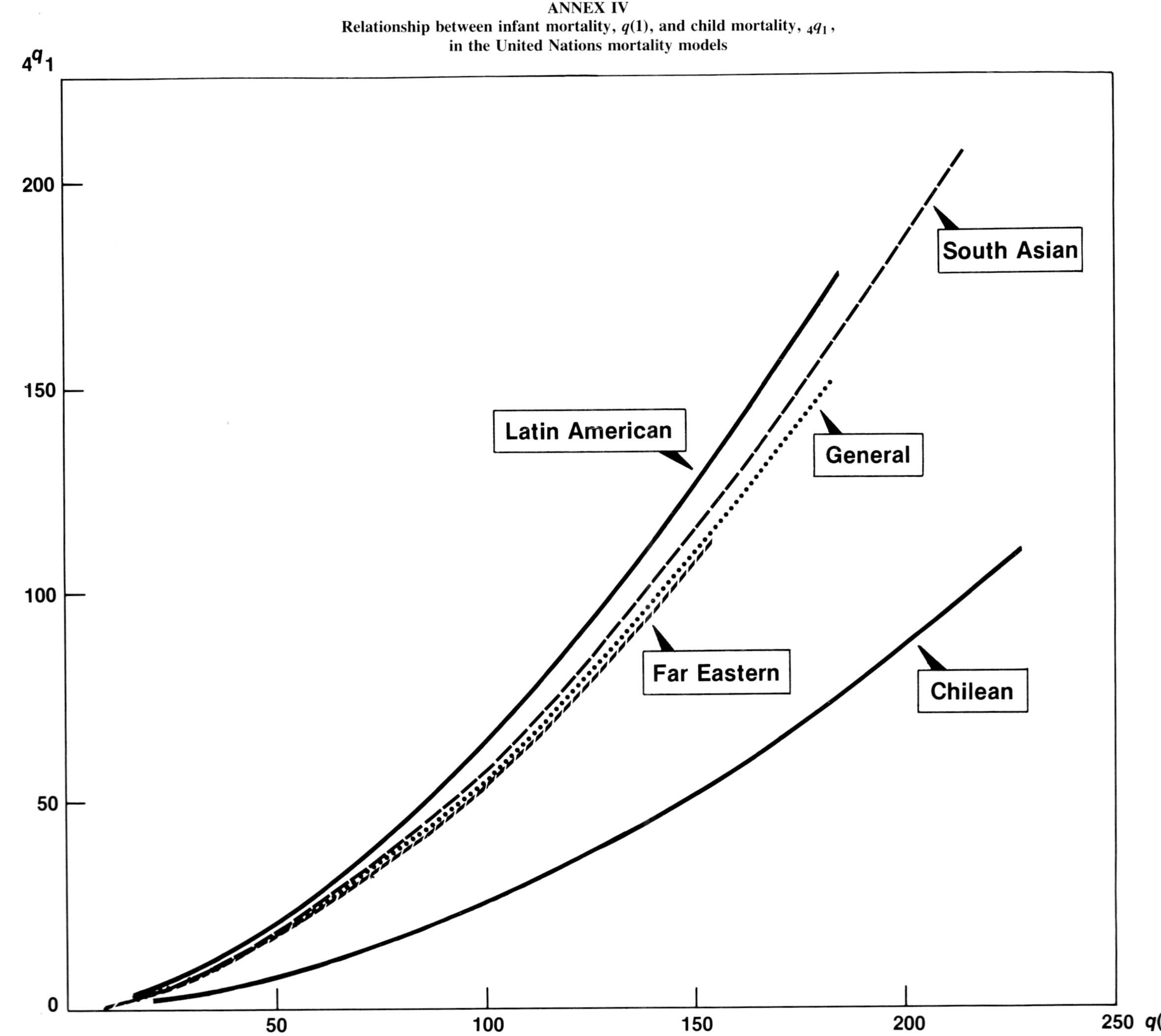

[1] For a description of how a life table is constructed in practice, see Henry S. Shryock, Jacob S. Siegel and others, *The Methods and Materials of Demography* (Washington, D.C., U.S. Department of Commerce, 1973), vol. 2, pp. 429-461.

[2] To understand the type of data collected, it is recommended that the analyst refer to the questionnaire used to gather the data and even to the instructions given to interviewers or enumerators. Unfortunately, those documents are often not published together with the tabulations of the data. However, whenever they are accessible, it is recommended that the analyst indicate how the information on children ever born and surviving was collected when presenting the results obtained from applying the Brass method.

[3] See, for instance, Alejandro Aguirre and Allan G. Hill, "Childhood mortality estimates using the preceding birth technique: some applications and extensions", CPS Research Paper 87-2 (Centre for Population Studies, London School of Hygiene and Tropical Medicine, September 1987).

[4] See, for instance, A. G. Hill and others, "L'enquête pilote sur la mortalité aux jeunes âges dans cinq maternités de la ville de Bamako, Mali", in *Estimation de la mortalité du jeune enfant (0-5) pour guider les actions de santé dans les pays en développement. Séminaire INSERM*, vol. 145, 107-130 (Paris, 1985); and Alejandro Aguirre and Allan G. Hill, *op. cit;* W. Brass and S. Macrae, "Childhood mortality estimated from reports on previous births given by mothers at the time of a maternity: I. Preceding-births technique", *Asian and Pacific Census Forum,* vol. 11, No. 2 (November 1984); and Miguel Irigoyen and Sonia M. Mychaszula, "Estimación de la mortalidad infantil mediante el método del hijo previo: Aplicación en el Hospital Rural de Junín de los Andes", paper presented at the IUSSP Seminar on Collection and Processing of Demographic Data in Latin America, Santiago, 23-27 May 1988.

[5] See Irigoyen and Mychaszula, *op. cit.,* and Aguirre and Hill, *op. cit.*

[6] Brass and Macrae, *op. cit.,* p. 7.

$B(i)$	number of births in a given year to women in age group i
$_nd_x$	number of deaths between exact ages x and $x + n$
$D(i)$	proportion of children dead
e_x	expectation of life at exact age x
e_0	expectation of life at birth
i	age group of mother or age group of women (see table 3 for the correspondence between different values of i and specific age groups)
$l(x)$	number of survivors to exact age x
$_nL_x$	number of person-years lived between exact ages x and $x + n$
$_nm_x$	age-specific mortality rate
$mp(i)$	midpoint in years of age group i (used in calculating the mean age at maternity)
M	mean age at maternity
$P(i)$	average parity of women in age group i
$_nq_x$	probability of dying between exact ages x and $x + n$
$q(x)$	probability of dying between birth and exact age x
$q(1)$	infant mortality
$_1q_0$	infant mortality
$_5q_0$	under-five mortality
$q(5)$	under-five mortality
$_4q_1$	child mortality
$t(i)$	reference date

age-specific death rate: See *age-specific mortality rate.*

age-specific mortality rate: Number of deaths of persons aged x to $x + n$ per person-year lived by the population in that age group. Usually denoted by $_nm_x$.

average parity: Average number of children ever born per woman. Denoted by $P(i)$.

birth interval: The time elapsed between the births of any two consecutive children of a given women.

child mortality: The probability of dying between exact ages 1 and 4. Denoted by $_4q_1$. The equation relating $_4q_1$ to infant and under-five mortality is

$$_4q_1 = (q(5) - q(1)) \neq (1.0 - q(1))$$

cohort: A group of persons experiencing the same event during a given period. A birth cohort is the group of persons born during the same period (usually a year).

exact age: A person's age at the exact moment of reaching a certain age, i.e., not one day younger or older than that age.

expectation of life at age x: Average number of additional years that a person aged x is expected to live under the mortality conditions represented by a life table. Denoted by e_x.

expectation of life at birth: Average number of years that a newly born person is expected to live under the mortality conditions represented by a life table. Denoted by e_0.

fertility history: Set of dates of birth and, where appropriate, dates of death of all children borne by a woman.

hypothetical cohort: A construct representing a cohort that does not really exist. Most life tables represent the effects of mortality on hypothetical birth cohorts (see *cohort*).

infant: Person under age 1.

infant mortality: The probability of dying between birth and exact age 1. Denoted by $q(1)$ or by $_1q_0$.

infant mortality rate: The number of deaths of children aged 0 to 1 per person-year lived by those children. Denoted by $_1m_0$.

life table: The demographer's way of representing the effects of mortality. It consists of several sets of numbers, or functions, each representing one particular aspect of the incidence of mortality in a population.

mean age at maternity: The mean age of mothers at the birth of a group of children, usually those born in a given year. It is denoted by M and used in the application of the Palloni-Heligman version of the Brass method.

not-stated parity: Refers to women who do not report the number of children they have had.

parity: Number of children ever borne by a woman. Abortions and still-births are not counted.

parity ratio: The ratio of average parities for women in different age groups. Those used in the Brass method are $P(1)/P(2)$ and $P(2)/P(3)$.

proportion of children dead: The ratio of children dead to children ever born, usually calculated for different age groups of women. Denoted by $D(i)$.

radix: Initial number of births in a life table subject to the mortality conditions it represents. The radix is denoted by $1(0)$ and it is usually 100,000.

reference date: Date to which estimates of mortality in childhood refer. Expressed in number of years before the survey or census gathering the basic information. Denoted by $t(i)$.

reproductive age: The age-span during which women are able to conceive. The reproductive-age span is usually set to range between exact ages 15 and 50, that is, 15-49 in completed years.

robustness: Characteristic of estimates that are not greatly affected by deviations from the assumptions upon which their derivation is based. An estimate is said to be robust to assumption *A*, when deviations from that particular assumption bring about only small changes in the value of the estimate.

sex ratio at birth: Average number of male births per female birth. It varies between 1.03 and 1.08 male births per female birth.

standard five-year age groups: Age groups of the following type: 0-4, 5-9, 10-14, 15-19 etc.

under-five mortality: The probability of dying between birth and exact age 5. Denoted by $q(5)$ or $_5q_0$.

weighted average: The weighted average A of quantities $Z(1)$, $Z(2), \ldots, Z(n)$, using weights $W(1)$, $W(2), \ldots, W(n)$, is calculated as follows:

$$A = \frac{\sum_{j=1}^{n} W(j)Z(j)}{\sum_{j=1}^{n} W(j)}$$

Aguirre, A., and A. G. Hill (1987). Childhood mortality estimates using the preceding birth technique: some applications and extensions. CPS Research Paper 87-2. Centre for Population Studies, London School of Hygiene and Tropical Medicine.

Bangladesh, Census Commission (1977). Report on the 1974 Bangladesh Retrospective Survey of Fertility and Mortality. Dacca.

Brass, W. (1964). Uses of census and survey data for the estimation of vital rates. Paper prepared for the African Seminar on Vital Statistics, Addis Ababa, 14-19 December 1964. United Nations document E/CN.14/CAS.4/VS/7.

Brass, W., and S. Macrae (1984). Childhood mortality estimated from reports on previous births given by mothers at the time of a maternity: I. Preceding-births technique. *Asian and Pacific Census Forum,* vol. 11, No. 2 (November).

Bucht, Birgitta (1988). Adequacy of aggregate child survival data for estimating mortality levels and trends. Paper presented at the IUSSP Seminar on Collection and Processing of Demographic Data in Latin America, Santiago, 23-27 May 1988.

Coale, A. J., and P. Demeny, with B. Vaughan (1983). *Regional Model Life Tables and Stable Populations.* 2nd ed. New York: Academic Press.

Coale, A. J., and T. J. Trussell (1978). Estimating the time to which Brass estimates apply. Annex I to Fine-tuning Brass-type mortality estimates with data on ages of surviving children, by S. H. Preston and A. Palloni. *Population Bulletin of the United Nations,* No. 10. Sales No. E.78.XIII.6.

Feeney, G. (1980). Estimating infant mortality trends from child survivorship data. *Population Studies,* vol. 34, No. 1.

Hill, A. G., and others (1985). L'enqute pilote sur la mortalité aux jeunes âges dans cinq maternités de la ville de Bamako, Mali. In *Estimation de la mortalité du jeune enfant (0-5) pour guider les actions de santé dans les pays en développement.* Séminaire INSERM, vol. 145. Paris.

Palloni, A., and L. Heligman (1986). Re-estimation of structural parameters to obtain estimates of mortality in developing countries. *Population Bulletin of the United Nations,* No. 18. Sales No. E.85.XIII.6.

Trussell, T. J. (1975). A re-estimation of the multiplying factors for the Brass technique for determining childhood survivorship rates. *Population Studies,* vol. 29, No. 1, pp. 97-108.

United Nations (1982). *Model Life Tables for Developing Countries.* Population Studies, No. 77. Sales No. E.81.XIII.7.

________ (1983a). Infant mortality: world estimates and projections, 1950-2025. *Population Bulletin of the United Nations,* No. 14. Sales No. E.82.XIII.6.

________ (1983b). *Manual X: Indirect Techniques for Demographic Estimation.* Population Studies, No. 81. Sales No. E.83.XIII.2.

________ (1986). *World Population Prospects: Estimates and Projections as Assessed in 1984,* Population Studies, No. 98. Sales No. E.85.XIII.3.

________ (1988). *Mortality of Children under Age 5: World Estimates and Projections, 1950-2025.* Population Studies, No. 105. Sales No. E.88.XIII.4.

United Nations Children's Fund (UNICEF) (1986). *Statistics on Children in UNICEF Assisted Countries.*

________ (1987a). *The State of the World's Children, 1987.* Oxford and New York: Oxford University Press.

________ (1987b). *Statistics on Children in UNICEF Assisted Countries.*

________ (1988a). *The State of the World's Children, 1988.* Oxford and New York: Oxford University Press.

________(1988b). *Statistics on Children in UNICEF Assisted Countries.*

كيفية الحصول على منشورات الأمم المتحدة

يمكن الحصول على منشورات الأمم المتحدة من المكتبات ودور التوزيع في جميع أنحاء العالم . استعلم عنها من المكتبة
التي تتعامل معها أو اكتب إلى : الأمم المتحدة ، قسم البيع في نيويورك أو في جنيف .

如何购取联合国出版物

联合国出版物在全世界各地的书店和经售处均有发售。请向书店询问或写信到纽约或日内瓦的
联合国销售组。

HOW TO OBTAIN UNITED NATIONS PUBLICATIONS

United Nations publications may be obtained from bookstores and distributors throughout the
world. Consult your bookstore or write to: United Nations, Sales Section, New York or Geneva.

COMMENT SE PROCURER LES PUBLICATIONS DES NATIONS UNIES

Les publications des Nations Unies sont en vente dans les librairies et les agences dépositaires
du monde entier. Informez-vous auprès de votre libraire ou adressez-vous à : Nations Unies,
Section des ventes, New York ou Genève.

КАК ПОЛУЧИТЬ ИЗДАНИЯ ОРГАНИЗАЦИИ ОБЪЕДИНЕННЫХ НАЦИЙ

Издания Организации Объединенных Наций можно купить в книжных магазинах
и агентствах во всех районах мира. Наводите справки об изданиях в вашем книжном
магазине или пишите по адресу: Организация Объединенных Наций, Секция по
продаже изданий, Нью-Йорк или Женева.

COMO CONSEGUIR PUBLICACIONES DE LAS NACIONES UNIDAS

Las publicaciones de las Naciones Unidas están en venta en librerías y casas distribuidoras en
todas partes del mundo. Consulte a su librero o diríjase a: Naciones Unidas, Sección de Ventas,
Nueva York o Ginebra.

Litho in United Nations, New York   01900   United Nations publication
89-40940—April 1990—4,075   Sales No. E.89.XIII.9
ISBN 92-1-151183-6   ST/ESA/SER.A/107

Department of International Economic and Social Affairs

ST/ESA/SER.A/107

Population Studies No. 107

QFIVE - UNITED NATIONS PROGRAM FOR CHILD MORTALITY ESTIMATION

A microcomputer program to accompany the Step-by-Step Guide to the Estimation of Child Mortality

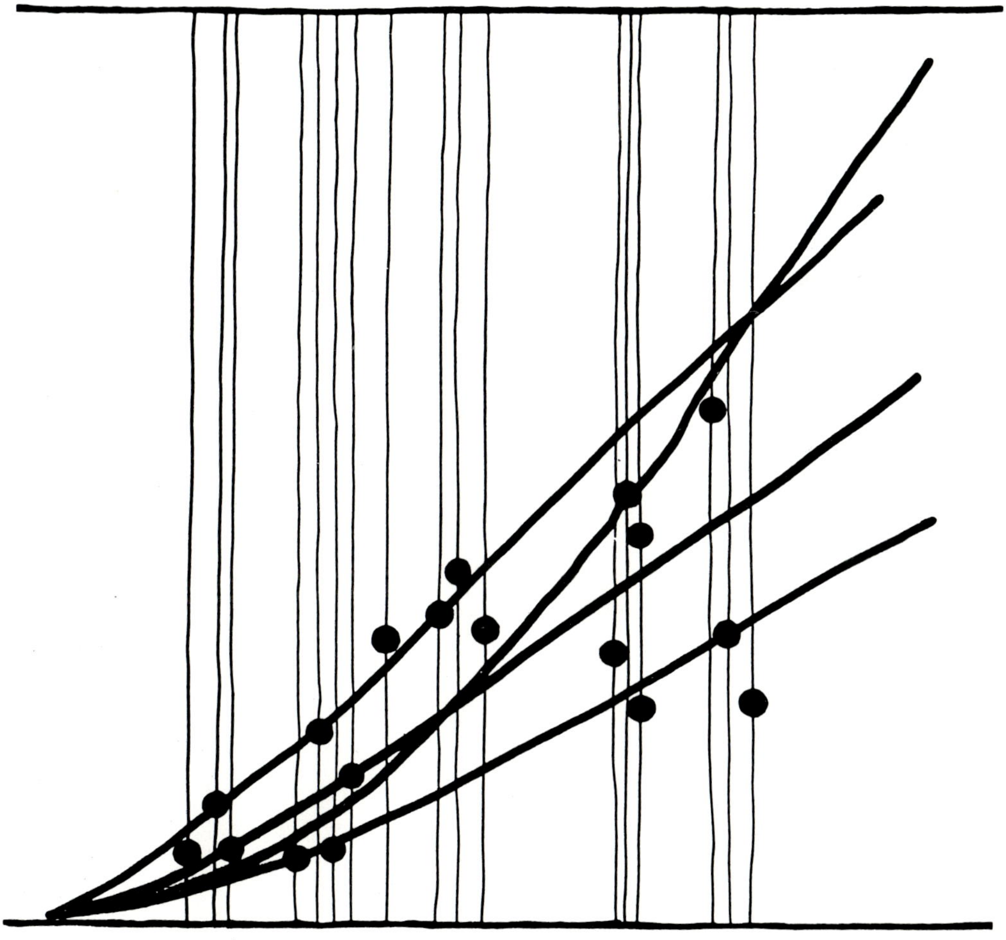

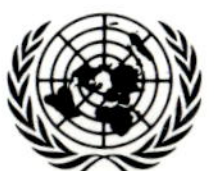

United Nations New York, 1990

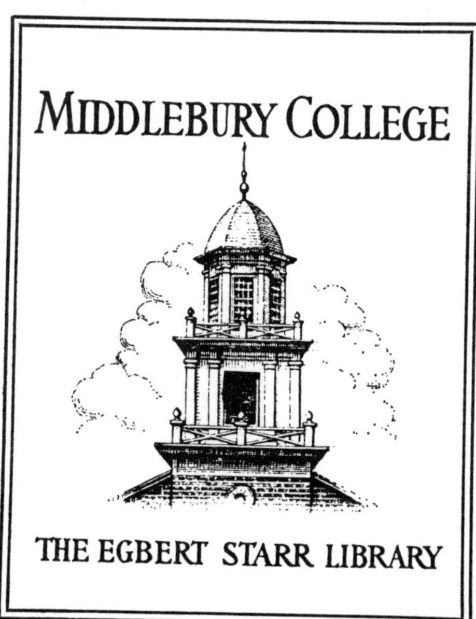
MIDDLEBURY COLLEGE
THE EGBERT STARR LIBRARY

CONTENTS

		Page
INTRODUCTION		1
I.	HARDWARE REQUIREMENTS AND INSTALLATION	3
	A. Hardware requirements	3
	B. Backup and installation	3
II.	USING QFIVE	4
	A. Getting started	4
	B. Moving through the screens	4
	C. The main menu	5
	Option 1. Enter or modify input data	5
	Option 2. Run QFIVE	10
	Option 3. Print, view, copy or delete a data set	11
	Option D. Change drive specifications	15
	Option H. Help	16
	Option X. Exit QFIVE	16
III.	DESCRIPTION OF THE OUTPUT	17

INTRODUCTION

These are instructions for the use of QFIVE, a computer program to estimate mortality in childhood. The program has been prepared to accompany the *Step-by-Step Guide to the Estimation of Child Mortality*. QFIVE produces estimates of infant mortality (the probability of dying between birth and exact age 1), child mortality (the probability of dying between exact ages 1 and 5) and under-five mortality (the probability of dying between birth and exact age 5) by applying the two versions of the Brass method described in the *Guide:* the Trussell version, which is based on the Coale-Demeny model life tables, and the Palloni-Heligman version, based on the United Nations model life tables for developing countries.

Anyone familiar with the contents of the *Guide,* even the inexperienced computer user, should find QFIVE simple to use. Its design follows that of *Mortpak-Lite, the United Nations Software Package for Mortality Measurement: Interactive Software for the IBM-PC and Compatibles.*[a] The chapters that follow describe the hardware requirements of QFIVE, the use of the program itself and the output it produces. Self-explanatory screens guide the user during each application, making QFIVE a useful self-teaching tool.

Knowledge of the estimation methodology, however, is essential. Appropriate use and interpretation of the estimates yielded by QFIVE demand a good understanding of the methods applied and their limitations. The user is referred to the *Guide* for an in-depth discussion of these topics.

The input required for QFIVE is described in the *Guide* for the different versions of the Brass method. It consists mainly of the number of children ever born and surviving, or dead, classified by age of mother and the number of women classified by age. In order to minimize hand calculations in the preparation of input data, QFIVE accepts as input several data combinations that permit the calculation of the basic information needed to apply the method.

The Population Division of the United Nations Secretariat would welcome any comments on the performance of QFIVE that might help improve future software development activities. For further information concerning QFIVE, please contact the Director, Population Division, United Nations, New York, New York 10017.

---

[a] United Nations publication, Sales No. E.88.XIII.2.

I. HARDWARE REQUIREMENTS AND INSTALLATION

QFIVE 1.0 can run on an IBM-PC–compatible microcomputer equipped with MS-DOS, version 2.1 or later, and a random access memory of 300K or more. Although, strictly speaking, only one floppy-disk drive is needed to run the program, it is easier to use when a hard disk or two floppy-disk drives are available. A math co-processor or graphics adaptor is not necessary.

The output of the program can either be viewed on the screen or be printed. To print the output, a printer with an IBM Graphics or Proprinter set-up is required. The output will be printed in compressed mode, which will be set automatically by QFIVE, using standard IBM printer control codes.

B. Backup and installation

QFIVE is stored on one diskette, which also contains two sample input files.

Before installation, it is recommended that you write-protect and make a backup copy of your QFIVE diskette. Put the original away for safekeeping and work only with your backup. If your system has a hard disk, installation of the QFIVE program on the hard disk will automatically create a backup. In systems with two floppy-disk drives and no hard disk, the procedure that follows can be used to make backups. Press **ENTER** after each DOS command.

STEP 1. Change the prompt line to **A>**

STEP 2. Insert the DOS diskette in drive A and format a blank diskette in drive B by typing the DOS command
A>FORMAT B:

STEP 3. When the formatting process is completed, copy the **COMMAND** command to the diskette in drive B by typing
A>COPY COMMAND.COM B:

STEP 4. Insert the original (write-protected) QFIVE diskette in drive A and the newly formatted diskette in drive B; then copy all files from drive A to drive B by typing the DOS command
A>COPY A:*.* B:

Keep the original QFIVE diskette in a safe place. Always work with the copy.

If your system has a hard disk, it is convenient to copy the contents of the QFIVE diskette onto the hard disk. To do so, follow the procedure below. Press **ENTER** after each DOS command.

STEP 1. Change the prompt line to **C>** by typing **C:**

STEP 2. Make a new subdirectory called QFIVE by typing the DOS command
C>MD QFIVE

(You can use any valid directory name instead of QFIVE.)

STEP 3. Enter that subdirectory by typing the DOS command
C>CD QFIVE

STEP 4. Insert the QFIVE diskette in drive A, and copy all files from that diskette to the QFIVE directory on the hard disk by typing the DOS command
C>COPY A:*.* C:

II. USING QFIVE

This chapter describes the QFIVE interface, explains how to start QFIVE, how to enter data and how to run the program. Chapter III describes the output.

A. GETTING STARTED

To start QFIVE on a hard-disk system, change to the QFIVE subdirectory by typing the DOS command

C > CD \QFIVE

and pressing **ENTER.**

At the C > prompt, type

C > QFIVE

and press **ENTER.**

On a one- or two-drive system, put the QFIVE program diskette into drive A, and at the A > prompt-type

A > QFIVE

and press **ENTER.**

These commands start the operation of QFIVE. The screen displays a welcome, followed by the QFIVE copyright notice. Press any key to get to the main menu. The last line on the main menu screen indicates the existing drive specifications—that is, it specifies the drives where QFIVE expects to find or allocate different files. Those specifications must agree with your program set-up. To change them, select option D and press **ENTER.** For instructions, refer to the section on main menu option D, below.

B. MOVING THROUGH THE SCREENS

QFIVE has a menu-based interface built around a main menu. The main menu offers primary options; each option moves the user through a series of screens on which the user provides certain pieces of information that determine the next screen that will appear.

Screen change is initiated by pressing either the **ENTER** key in response to a question or an F-key (function key). The function keys accepted by QFIVE and their definitions are as follows:

F1	Presents help screens
F2	Returns user to main menu
F3	Moves user to utility menu (to print, view, copy or delete data sets)
F4	Lists files on a specified drive
F5	Copies files on a specified drive into the currently active worksheet during edit
F9	Runs the program directly from the worksheet
F10	Saves data in the active worksheet and returns to the main menu

Active function keys are indicated at the bottom of the screen. < **ENT** > following the indicated function key means that the **ENTER** key must be pressed after pressing the function key.

QFIVE is built around the following main menu:

```
------------------------   QFIVE   --------------------------
----- United Nations Program for Child Mortality Estimation  -----

                        MAIN MENU

            (1) Enter or modify input data
            (2) Run QFIVE
            (3) Print, view, copy or delete a data set
            (D) Change drive specifications
            (H) Help
            (X) Exit QFIVE


        Please select option and press ENTER:




    Drive specifications      QFIVE : C    INPUT : C    OUTPUT : C
```

The main menu contains six options, each of which will be discussed in turn.

Main menu option 1. Enter or modify input data

Selection of option 1 will move the user to a screen asking for the name of the data set to be edited. If a new data set is being created, the user should assign it a new name according to DOS conventions: up to eight characters before the period and an optional extension of three characters after the period. Names containing more characters will be truncated to eight and three characters respectively.

If an existing data set is being modified, enter its name. Note that pressing **F4** followed by the **ENTER** key will provide a list of all files on the designated input drive.

After the data set name has been entered, the first page of a two-page worksheet will appear, and the user will be asked for the following information:

Label	Up to 72 characters describing the input data. The label will be printed as a header on each page of output.
Month	A number from 1 to 12 indicating the month of enumeration. If the data collection took place over several months, provide the central one.
Year	The year of enumeration.
Sex	A number from 1 to 3 indicating the sex of the children whose mortality is being estimated.
Mean age at maternity	The value of M needed for the application of the Palloni-Heligman version of the Brass method (see step 3(a) in chapter V of the *Guide*). If the data necessary to calculate M are not available and a value is not given for M, the program will use 27.0 as the default value.
Type of data	A number from 1 to 5 indicating the type of data to be used as input. QFIVE admits several data combinations as input, as explained below.

As described in chapter II of the *Guide,* three pieces of information are necessary to estimate mortality in childhood using the Brass method: (1) the number of children ever born classified by age group of mother, (2) the number of children dead classified by age group of mother and (3) the total number of women classified by age group. Since the sources of such data often do not contain tabulations of the number of children ever born and dead *per se,* QFIVE accepts as input different data combinations from which the required pieces of information can be derived.

The data combinations admitted, which are also defined on the screen, are as follows:

1.   Number of children ever born, number of children surviving and total number of women classified by age group.

2.   Number of children ever born, number of children dead and total number of women classified by age group.

3.   Number of children surviving, number of children dead and total number of women classified by age group.

4.   Average parity by age group of women and the proportion of children dead by age group of women. Average parity is the ratio of the number of children ever born to the number of women. The proportion of children dead is the ratio of the number of children dead to the number of children ever born.

5.   Average parity and average number of children surviving by age group of women. Children surviving per woman is the ratio of the number of children surviving to the number of women.

The type of information required for input options 4 and 5 is often the only type available from the secondary sources that do not present the raw data needed for the application of the Brass method. These options should be used only if the raw data are not available, since rounding and other types of errors could have been introduced in the calculations to obtain the average numbers.

The necessary information should be typed in and **ENTER** or a cursor key should be pressed after each item has been completed. Make sure that all items are typed according to the specifications provided on the screen. An example of a properly completed first page is provided below.

```
                    Q F I V E      Data Entry      (Page 1 of 2)

LABEL: BANGLADESH, 1974 RETROSPECTIVE SURVEY


              Month (1 - 12) ..........................   3
              Year (4 digits) ........................ 1974
              Sex (1=Male, 2=Female, 3=Both) ..........   3
              Mean Age at Maternity (Default 27.0).....27.07
              Type of data (choose 1-5, below)........   1


                            Data Types

        1 = Number of women, children ever born and children surviving
        2 = Number of women, children ever born and children dead
        3 = Number of women, children surviving and children dead
        4 = Average parity and proportion of children dead
        5 = Average parity and children surviving per woman


    F1 - Help    F2 - Main Menu    F5 - Copy    F9 - Run    F10 - Save  (PgUp/PgDn)
```

Once the "Type of data" entry has been provided, the second page of the input worksheet can be obtained by pressing the **PgUp** or **PgDn** key. The headings appearing on the second page will vary according to the "Type of data" selected. Entries can be made in the worksheet by typing each number and pressing **ENTER** once the entry is completed. For purposes of illustration, the screens below show how the second page looks according to the "Type of data" selected.

Type of data = 1

```
            Q F I V E     Data Entry     (Page 2 of 2)


    ---------     ---------     ---------     ---------
    Age Group      Number      Number of     Number of
       of            of         Children      Children
      Women         Women      Ever Born     Surviving
    ---------     ---------     ---------     ---------
     15 - 19       3014706       1160919        945554
     20 - 24       2653155       4901382       3903998
     25 - 29       2607009       9085852       7147897
     30 - 34       2015663       9910256       7649060
     35 - 39       1771680      10384001       7893833
     40 - 44       1479575       9164329       6749306
     45 - 49       1135129       6905673       4946129




F1 - Help    F2 - Main Menu    F5 - Copy    F9 - Run    F10 - Save   (PgUp/PgDn)
```

Type of data = 2

```
            Q F I V E     Data Entry     (Page 2 of 2)


    ---------     ---------     ---------     ---------
    Age Group      Number      Number of     Number of
       of            of         Children      Children
      Women         Women      Ever Born        Dead
    ---------     ---------     ---------     ---------
     15 - 19       3014706       1160919        215365
     20 - 24       2653155       4901382        997384
     25 - 29       2607009       9085852       1937955
     30 - 34       2015663       9910256       2261196
     35 - 39       1771680      10384001       2490168
     40 - 44       1479575       9164329       2415023
     45 - 49       1135129       6905673       1959544




F1 - Help    F2 - Main Menu    F5 - Copy    F9 - Run    F10 - Save   (PgUp/PgDn)
```

Type of data = 3

```
          Q F I V E     Data Entry    (Page 2 of 2)


     ---------    ---------    ---------    ---------
     Age Group      Number     Number of    Number of
        of            of        Children     Children
       Women         Women     Surviving      Dead
     ---------    ---------    ---------    ---------
       15 - 19      3014706       945554       215365
       20 - 24      2653155      3903998       997384
       25 - 29      2607009      7147897      1937955
       30 - 34      2015663      7649060      2261196
       35 - 39      1771680      7893833      2490168
       40 - 44      1479575      6749306      2415023
       45 - 49      1135129      4946129      1959544



 F1 - Help    F2 - Main Menu    F5 - Copy    F9 - Run    F10 - Save    (PgUp/PgDn)
```

Type of data = 4

```
          Q F I V E     Data Entry    (Page 2 of 2)


     ---------              -------         -----------
     Age Group              Average         Proportion
        of                  Parity          of Children
       Woman                                   Dead
     ---------              -------         -----------
       15 - 19              0.3851            0.1855
       20 - 24              1.8474            0.2035
       25 - 29              3.4852            0.2133
       30 - 34              4.9166            0.2282
       35 - 39              5.8611            0.2398
       40 - 44              6.1940            0.2635
       45 - 49              6.0836            0.2838



 F1 - Help    F2 - Main Menu    F5 - Copy    F9 - Run    F10 - Save    (PgUp/PgDn)
```

$$\text{Type of data} = 5$$

```
                Q  F  I  V  E      Data Entry     (Page 2 of 2)


            ----------              -------            -------------
            Age Group               Average           Average No.
               of                   Parity            of Children
             Woman                                    Surviving
            ----------              -------            -------------
              15 - 19               0.3851                0.3136
              20 - 24               1.8474                1.4715
              25 - 29               3.4852                2.7423
              30 - 34               4.9166                3.7952
              35 - 39               5.8611                4.4568
              40 - 44               6.1940                4.5625
              45 - 49               6.0836                4.3578




   F1 - Help     F2 - Main Menu     F5 - Copy     F9 - Run     F10 - Save   (PgUp/PgDn)
```

Note that the data entries for input options 1, 2 and 3 must be in absolute numbers. Entries must have at most 10 figures. No commas should be used to separate them. Entries for options 4 and 5 can have at most four decimal places, and the decimal point must be indicated explicitly, as, for instance, in 1.8474.

The process of data input is straightforward. Cursor movement is restricted to valid input data fields and is controlled by keyboard keys. Whenever the cursor leaves a field, numeric data are right-justified. Definitions of the keys are as follows:

ENTER	This key moves the cursor to the next data field.
CURSOR (arrow)	These keys move the cursor left, right, up or down one position.
BACKSPACE	This key moves the cursor one position to the left and deletes the entered character.
RIGHT TAB	This key moves the cursor one field to the right.
LEFT TAB	This key (shift tab) moves the cursor one field to the left.
HOME	This key moves the cursor to the first position of the first data field on the page.
END	This key moves the cursor to the last non-blank character of the field plus one. If the last character is not blank, it moves the cursor to the last character of the field.
CTRL-END	Pressing these keys simultaneously erases all data from the current cursor position through the end of the field.
INSERT	From the point of the cursor, this key moves all data from within the field one position to the right.
DELETE	This key deletes the character at the cursor position. Data in the same field and to the right of the cursor moves left one position.
PgUp/PgDn	These keys are used for moving between the two pages of the worksheet.

The **F5** key, which appears on the screen on both pages of the worksheet, enables the user to copy data from a different file into the active worksheet.

Main menu option 2. Run QFIVE

To run QFIVE, the user can either press **F9** from the input worksheet or select option 2 from the main menu. The choice of option 2 leads to a screen requesting the name of the input file.

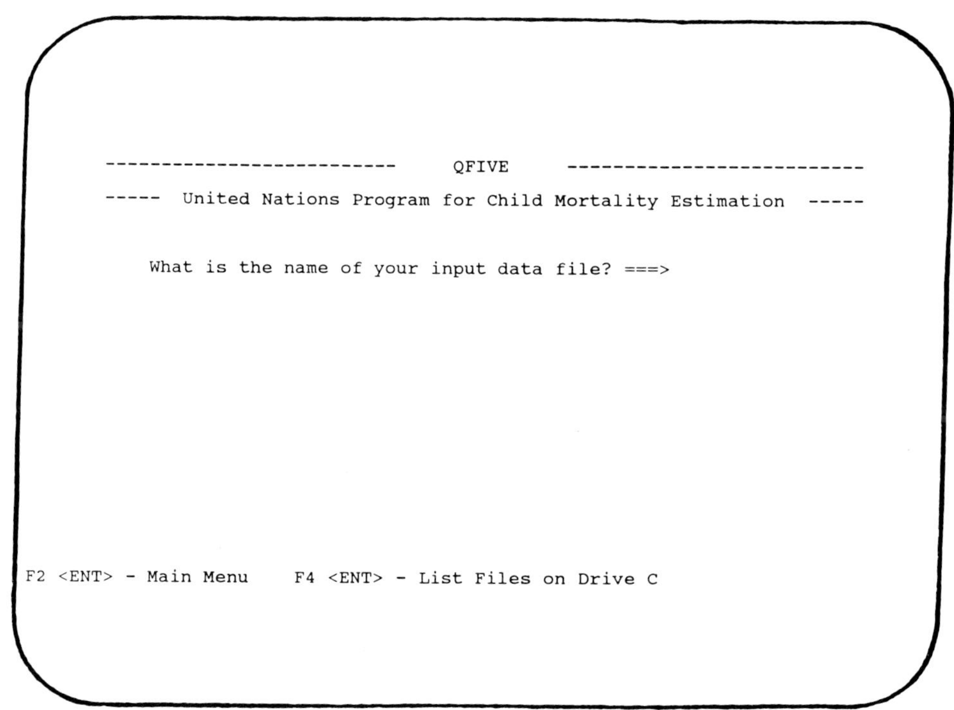

At the query, the user should provide the name of an existing input file. Two function keys are available at the bottom of the screen. The **F2** <ENT> key sequence returns the user to the main menu; the **F4** <ENT> key sequence displays a list of all files on the input data drive.

Pressing the **ENTER** key after entering the file name causes the program to run. When processing is complete, the screen shown at the top of page 11 (referred to as a utility menu) appears, allowing the user to route the output.

Option 1 sends the output to the printer. Make sure that the printer is on-line before selecting option 1. Before printing, the question "How many copies would you like?" appears on the screen. Any integer response is acceptable; there is no maximum number of copies. The default is 1. Printing will begin immediately.

Option 2 sends the output to the screen. It is usually a good idea to examine the output on the screen to ensure that it is correct before sending it to the printer or saving it on disk. After viewing the output on the screen, the user can return to the utility menu by pressing **F3** <ENT> and can then choose option 1 or 3, to print or save the output.

Option 3 saves the output on disk. The user is requested to provide the name of the output file to be saved. It should conform to DOS naming conventions. Typing the output file name and

```
------------------------- QFIVE -------------------------
----- United Nations Program for Child Mortality Estimation -----



                    Where would you like your output?

                        (1) Routed to the printer
                        (2) Viewed on the screen
                        (3) Saved on disk

            Please select option number and press ENTER:




F2 <ENT> - Main Menu
```

pressing **ENTER** copies the output file onto the output drive under the designated file name. Once this is completed, the user is returned to the utility menu.

Main menu option 3. Print, view, copy or delete a data set

This option allows the user to carry out common file-handling activities without returning to DOS. Selection of option 3 yields the screen shown at the top of page 12.

Option 1 routes a file to the printer. Selection of option 1 calls forth a series of screens querying the user for characteristics of the file to be printed: whether it is an input or an output data set, the name of the data set and the number of copies desired (second illustration, page 12, and page 13).

Option 2 routes a file to the screen for viewing. As in the case of option 1, several queries about characteristics of the file will appear on the screen. Specifically, the user is asked: "Will you view on the screen an input or output data file?" and "What is the name of the data set you wish to view on the screen?" Often the output file wanted is the last one processed. This can be indicated by typing in **LAST OUTPUT.**

The user should note that this utility will print or display an input file using the format in which the data are stored on disk. To see the input data in worksheet format (i.e., with the appropriate headings), one must use option 1 of the main menu or print the first page of an output file.

```
------------------------  QFIVE  ------------------------
----- United Nations Program for Child Mortality Estimation  -----


                    ----------------------
                         UTILITY MENU
                    ----------------------

            (1)  Print
            (2)  View on the screen
            (3)  Copy
            (4)  Delete


        Please select option number and press ENTER:




F2 <ENT> - Main Menu
```

```
------------------------  QFIVE  ------------------------
----- United Nations Program for Child Mortality Estimation  -----



        Will you print an input or output data file?

            (1)  Input data   (from drive C)
            (2)  Output data  (from drive C)

        Please select option number and press ENTER:




F2 <ENT> - Main Menu     F3 <ENT> - Utility Menu
```

```
------------------------  QFIVE  ------------------------
-----  United Nations Program for Child Mortality Estimation  -----


   What is the name of the data set you wish to print?
   To print your last output, type LAST.OUTPUT
   For example: CHILD.DAT    ===>
```

F2 <ENT> - Main Menu F3 <ENT> - Utility Menu   F4 <ENT> - List Files on Drive C

```
------------------------  QFIVE  ------------------------
-----  United Nations Program for Child Mortality Estimation  -----



            How many copies would you like? 1
```

F2 <ENT> - Main Menu   F3 <ENT> - Utility Menu

The following screen displays an output file as viewed on the screen.

```
INPUT DATA FOR BANGLADESH, 1974 RETROSPECTIVE SURVEY
BOTH SEXES
ENUMERATION DATE: MAR 1974


---------   ---------   ---------   ---------
Age Group    Number     Number of   Number of
   of          of       Children    Children
 Women       Women      Ever Born   Surviving
---------   ---------   ---------   ---------
  15-19     3014706.     1160919.     945554.
  20-24     2653155.     4901382.    3903998.
  25-29     2607009.     9085852.    7147897.
  30-34     2015663.     9910256.    7649060.
  35-39     1771680.    10384001.    7893833.
  40-44     1479575.     9164329.    6749306.
  45-49     1135129.     6905673.    4946129.

INDIRECT ESTIMATION OF EARLY AGE MORTALITY FOR BANGLADESH, 1974 RETRO
BOTH SEXES
ENUMERATION DATE: MAR 1974
======================================================================
F2 - Main Menu   F3 - Utility Menu   Use cursors to scroll ===> PAGE
```

When viewing a file, the user can return at any time to the main menu by pressing **F2** <ENT> or to the utility menu by pressing **F3** <ENT>.

Because of screen size, only part of a file can be seen at one time. The cursor keys are used to scroll the screen in order to view different parts of a file. The cursor functions are:

RIGHT CURSOR   Exhibits data to the right of the screen.

LEFT CURSOR   Exhibits data to the left of the screen.

DOWN CURSOR   Exhibits data below the screen.

UP CURSOR   Exhibits data above the screen.

The extent of scrolling is determined by the user and is indicated at the bottom right-hand corner of the screen. Scrolling is always pre-set to "page". The extent of scrolling can be changed by pressing one of the keys indicated below:

M   Indicates "maximum". Depending on the cursor key pressed, data at the right, left, top or bottom margin are brought into view.

P   Indicates "page". The displayed data file is moved in the indicated direction a "full page"—that is, up to 23 lines or up to 80 columns, depending on the cursor key activated. Scrolling is always pre-set to **P**.

1 through 9   Entering an integer between 1 and 9 sets the scrolling to that number of lines or columns.

Option 3 allows the user to make copies of an input or output file (data set) on the same disk drive. This utility may be used, for example, to make a backup copy of a data set before modifying its contents. Before copying, the user must provide information on file characteristics by answering the queries: "What is the name of the data set you wish to copy?" and "In what data set would you like to save the copy?" If the data set already has a name, the user will be given the option of choosing another name for the backup copy or using the existing name. If the existing name is used and the data are modified, the original data will be destroyed.

Option 4 allows the user to delete files. The user must indicate whether an input or output data set is being deleted (only if input and output data sets reside on different disk drives) and the name of the data set to be deleted. Before the file is deleted, the user is asked to confirm that the selected file is to be deleted.

Main menu option D. Change drive specifications

Option D specifies the disk drives for the QFIVE program and the input and output files. Drive specifications must be correct for QFIVE to work properly. In a hard-disk drive system, QFIVE should be installed in drive C. The input and output files can be stored in any combination of drive A, B or C. In a two-drive system, QFIVE may be assigned to drive A, and the input and output files to drive B. In a one-drive system, QFIVE and the input and output files have to be assigned to drive A.

When option D is selected, the following screen will appear.

```
------------------------  QFIVE   ------------------------
-----  United Nations Program for Child Mortality Estimation  -----

              DISK DRIVE INSTALLATION PROCEDURE

        On what disk drive is QFIVE?
        Drive C is the current selection.
        Select a,b,c,d or blank and press ENTER:


        On what disk drive would you like your input data?
        Drive C is the current selection.
        Select a,b,c,d or blank and press ENTER:


        On what disk drive would you like your output?
        Drive C is the current selection.
        Select a,b,c,d or blank and press ENTER:
```

Pressing **ENTER** without making an entry (a blank response) leaves the existing selection active.

After a selection has been made for all items, the user is asked to confirm the choices made.

```
------------------------  QFIVE   ------------------------
----- United Nations Program for Child Mortality Estimation  -----


                    -----------------
                        SUMMARY
                    -----------------

                    QFIVE  : C
                    INPUT  : C
                    OUTPUT : C


          Are these the correct disk drives (yes or no)?
```

A "yes" response sets the indicated drive specifications and returns the user to the main menu. A "no" response returns the user to the previous screen to respecify the necessary drives.

QFIVE updates the information on drive specifications so that the latest configuration will appear on the screen the next time the program is used.

Main menu option H. Help

Option H brings forth a text providing general instructions on using QFIVE. An application-specific help screen is also available within the data-entry worksheet.

Main menu option X. Exit QFIVE

Option X ends the QFIVE session, clears memory and returns the user to DOS.

III. DESCRIPTION OF THE OUTPUT

An example of QFIVE's printed output is displayed on pages 18-20. The output can only be described as comprehensive. Three pages are printed for each set of input data. The label, sex of children and enumeration date are printed at the top of each page. The first page gives the input data in worksheet format as they were entered on the screen, while the second and third pages show the estimates obtained.

The second page presents the estimates produced by the application of the Trussell version of the Brass method, while the third presents the equivalent estimates obtained using the Palloni-Heligman version. Both pages consist of an upper panel showing the average number of children ever born (average parity), the average number of children surviving, the reported proportions dead and the estimates of the probability of dying by age x, $q(x)$, yielded by the different versions of the Brass method using all available mortality models. Each $q(x)$ is accompanied by the corresponding $t(i)$, its time reference, expressed in number of years before the date of the survey or census.

The lower panel of each page presents three sets of estimates: $q(1)$, that is, the probability of dying between birth and exact age 1, also known as infant mortality; $_4q_1$, the probability of dying between exact ages 1 and 5, termed "child mortality" in the *Guide*; and $q(5)$, the probability of dying between birth and exact age 5, also called "under-five mortality". All those estimates are "common indices" to which the estimates of $q(x)$ shown in the upper panel were translated by using model life tables. As explained in the *Guide*, it is recommended that the user focus on the estimated set of $q(5)$ equivalents. The estimates of $q(1)$ and $_4q_1$ are given to make comparisons possible with estimates from other sources where infant mortality is often the only measure of mortality in childhood used. The reference dates are given with one decimal point to make it easier to plot the estimates on a graph.

Note that QFIVE produces estimates for all the life-table models presented in the *Guide*. As explained in chapter IV of the *Guide*, the Trussell version is based on the Coale-Demeny regional model life tables, which have four variants: North, South, East and West. The Palloni-Heligman version, on the other hand, uses the United Nations model life tables for developing countries, whose five variants are Latin American, Chilean, South Asian, Far Eastern and General. The user is therefore faced with at least nine different sets of estimates for each set of input data. As suggested in the *Guide*, the best way of comparing and evaluating those estimates is graphically, by plotting the $q(5)$ estimates, for instance, against their respective reference dates (see figures 12 and 13 in chapter VI of the *Guide*).

Often, the user will not have to consider the whole array of estimates produced by QFIVE. If, for example, the data necessary to estimate the mean age at maternity (M) are not available, the user may wish to ignore the estimates produced by the Palloni-Heligman version, which would depend on an arbitrary default value for that parameter. If, on the other hand, additional evidence suggests that the mortality pattern in a country is very close to that of the Chilean model, the Trussell estimates and those produced by all other United Nations models can be disregarded. For a further discussion on choice of model life table and interpretation of the estimates, see chapter VI of the *Guide*.

Although QFIVE probably provides more information than is strictly necessary for the estimation of child mortality, this feature gives it added flexibility and should make it possible to meet the needs of most users.

Example of the first page of the printed output:

```
INPUT DATA FOR BANGLADESH, 1974 RETROSPECTIVE SURVEY
BOTH SEXES
ENUMERATION DATE: MAR 1974


----------   ----------   ----------   ----------
Age Group      Number      Number of    Number of
   of            of        Children     Children
 Women         Women       Ever Born    Surviving
----------   ----------   ----------   ----------
   15-19      3014706.     1160919.      945554.
   20-24      2653155.     4901382.     3903998.
   25-29      2607009.     9085852.     7147897.
   30-34      2015663.     9910256.     7649060.
   35-39      1771680.    10384001.     7893833.
   40-44      1479575.     9164329.     6749306.
   45-49      1135129.     6905673.     4946129.
```

Example of the second page of the printed output:

```
INDIRECT ESTIMATION OF EARLY AGE MORTALITY FOR BANGLADESH, 1974 RETROSPECTIVE SURVEY
BOTH SEXES
ENUMERATION DATE: MAR 1974
==================================================================================================

            AVERAGE NO.                                        COALE-DEMENY MODELS
AGE OF        CHILDREN     PROPORTION   AGE                    (TRUSSELL EQUATIONS)
WOMAN     BORN  SURVIVING    DEAD        X        NORTH            SOUTH           EAST            WEST
                                               q(x)   t(x)     q(x)   t(x)     q(x)   t(x)     q(x)   t(x)
-------------------------------------------------------------------------------------------------------
15-19      .385     .314      .186        1      .177  ( 1.2)   .170  ( 1.2)   .187  ( 1.2)   .182  ( 1.2)
20-24     1.847    1.471      .203        2      .193  ( 2.6)   .203  ( 2.6)   .206  ( 2.6)   .204  ( 2.6)
25-29     3.485    2.742      .213        3      .197  ( 4.5)   .211  ( 4.6)   .211  ( 4.7)   .208  ( 4.7)
30-34     4.917    3.795      .228        5      .221  ( 6.7)   .230  ( 7.0)   .227  ( 7.1)   .227  ( 7.0)
35-39     5.861    4.456      .240       10      .248  ( 9.2)   .247  ( 9.6)   .245  ( 9.8)   .243  ( 9.6)
40-44     6.194    4.562      .264       15      .270  (11.8)   .266  (12.4)   .265  (12.7)   .264  (12.3)
45-49     6.084    4.357      .284       20      .285  (14.6)   .283  (15.5)   .283  (15.9)   .282  (15.2)


==================================================================================================
COALE-DEMENY:         NORTH                SOUTH                EAST                 WEST
-------------------------------------------------------------------------------------------------------
AGE OF           REFERENCE           REFERENCE           REFERENCE           REFERENCE
WOMAN            DATE     q          DATE     q          DATE     q          DATE     q
-------------------------------------------------------------------------------------------------------
INFANT MORTALITY RATE:  q(1)

15-19            1973.0  .177        1973.0  .170        1973.0  .187        1973.0  .182
20-24            1971.7  .151        1971.6  .149        1971.6  .174        1971.6  .163
25-29            1969.7  .135        1969.6  .141        1969.5  .167        1969.6  .152
30-34            1967.5  .131        1967.2  .141        1967.1  .169        1967.2  .152
35-39            1965.1  .127        1964.6  .140        1964.4  .169        1964.6  .150
40-44            1962.4  .129        1961.8  .144        1961.5  .176        1961.9  .154
45-49            1959.6  .127        1958.7  .145        1958.3  .178        1959.0  .153


-------------------------------------------------------------------------------------------------------
PROBABILITY OF DYING BETWEEN AGES 1 AND 5:  q
                                           4 1
15-19            1973.0  .146        1973.0  .149        1973.0  .083        1973.0  .111
20-24            1971.7  .122        1971.6  .116        1971.6  .074        1971.6  .097
25-29            1969.7  .108        1969.6  .104        1969.5  .070        1969.6  .089
30-34            1967.5  .104        1967.2  .104        1967.1  .071        1967.2  .089
35-39            1965.1  .100        1964.6  .103        1964.4  .071        1964.6  .087
40-44            1962.4  .102        1961.8  .109        1961.5  .075        1961.9  .090
45-49            1959.6  .101        1958.7  .110        1958.3  .077        1959.0  .090


-------------------------------------------------------------------------------------------------------
PROBABILITY OF DYING BY AGE 5:  q(5)

15-19            1973.0  .297        1973.0  .294        1973.0  .254        1973.0  .273
20-24            1971.7  .254        1971.6  .248        1971.6  .235        1971.6  .244
25-29            1969.7  .228        1969.6  .230        1969.5  .225        1969.6  .228
30-34            1967.5  .221        1967.2  .230        1967.1  .227        1967.2  .227
35-39            1965.1  .214        1964.6  .229        1964.4  .228        1964.6  .224
40+44            1962.4  .218        1961.8  .237        1961.5  .238        1961.9  .230
45-49            1959.6  .215        1958.7  .239        1958.3  .241        1959.0  .229


==================================================================================================
NOTE: A q VALUE OF .999 DENOTES VALUE BELOW A LEVEL 1 MODEL LIFE TABLE
         "      .000       "        ABOVE A LEVEL 25              "
```

Example of the third page of the printed output:

INDIRECT ESTIMATION OF EARLY AGE MORTALITY FOR BANGLADESH, 1974 RETROSPECTIVE SURVEY
BOTH SEXES
ENUMERATION DATE: MAR 1974

AGE OF WOMAN	AVERAGE NO. CHILDREN BORN	SURVIVING	PROPORTION DEAD	AGE x	LATIN AM q(x)	t(x)	CHILEAN q(x)	t(x)	SO ASIAN q(x)	t(x)	FAR EAST q(x)	t(x)	GENERAL q(x)	t(x)
								UNITED NATIONS MODELS (PALLONI-HELIGMAN EQUATIONS)						
15-19	.385	.314	.186	1	.179	(1.1)	.199	(1.3)	.179	(1.1)	.183	(1.2)	.181	(1.1)
20-24	1.847	1.471	.203	2	.207	(2.5)	.215	(2.6)	.209	(2.5)	.206	(2.6)	.207	(2.5)
25-29	3.485	2.742	.213	3	.213	(4.3)	.217	(4.5)	.215	(4.4)	.211	(4.4)	.212	(4.3)
30-34	4.917	3.795	.228	5	.231	(6.5)	.231	(6.8)	.234	(6.6)	.227	(6.6)	.229	(6.5)
35-39	5.861	4.456	.240	10	.249	(8.9)	.243	(9.3)	.249	(9.1)	.243	(9.0)	.247	(8.9)
40-44	6.194	4.562	.264	15	.262	(11.7)	.264	(12.1)	.269	(12.0)	.262	(11.6)	.262	(11.7)
45-49	6.084	4.357	.284	20	.284	(15.3)	.283	(15.7)	.286	(15.9)	.283	(14.9)	.284	(15.2)

MEAN AGE AT MATERNITY = 27.07

UNITED NATIONS:	LATIN AM		CHILEAN		SO ASIAN		FAR EAST		GENERAL	
AGE OF WOMAN	REFERENCE DATE	q	REFERENCE DATE	q	REFERENCE DATE	q	REFERENCE DATE	q	REFERENCE DATE	q

INFANT MORTALITY RATE: q(1)

AGE OF WOMAN	LATIN AM DATE	q	CHILEAN DATE	q	SO ASIAN DATE	q	FAR EAST DATE	q	GENERAL DATE	q
15-19	1973.1	.179	1972.9	.199	1973.1	.179	1973.0	.999	1973.1	.181
20-24	1971.7	.155	1971.6	.185	1971.7	.157	1971.6	.999	1971.7	.160
25-29	1969.9	.142	1969.7	.176	1969.8	.146	1969.8	.148	1969.9	.147
30-34	1967.7	.138	1967.4	.175	1967.6	.143	1967.7	.144	1967.7	.143
35-39	1965.3	.135	1964.9	.174	1965.1	.142	1965.3	.139	1965.3	.140
40-44	1962.5	.136	1962.1	.179	1962.2	.148	1962.6	.139	1962.5	.141
45-49	1958.9	.138	1958.5	.180	1958.3	.150	1959.3	.134	1959.0	.142

PROBABILITY OF DYING BETWEEN AGES 1 AND 5: q
4 1

AGE OF WOMAN	LATIN AM DATE	q	CHILEAN DATE	q	SO ASIAN DATE	q	FAR EAST DATE	q	GENERAL DATE	q
15-19	1973.1	.166	1972.9	.086	1973.1	.152	1973.0	.999	1973.1	.148
20-24	1971.7	.131	1971.6	.075	1971.7	.123	1971.6	.999	1971.7	.120
25-29	1969.9	.114	1969.7	.068	1969.8	.108	1969.8	.103	1969.9	.105
30-34	1967.7	.108	1967.4	.068	1967.6	.105	1967.7	.098	1967.7	.100
35-39	1965.3	.105	1964.9	.067	1965.1	.104	1965.3	.092	1965.3	.097
40-44	1962.5	.105	1962.1	.071	1962.2	.111	1962.6	.092	1962.5	.097
45-49	1958.9	.109	1958.5	.071	1958.3	.114	1959.3	.088	1959.0	.098

PROBABILITY OF DYING BY AGE 5: q(5)

AGE OF WOMAN	LATIN AM DATE	q	CHILEAN DATE	q	SO ASIAN DATE	q	FAR EAST DATE	q	GENERAL DATE	q
15-19	1973.1	.316	1972.9	.268	1973.1	.304	1973.0	.999	1973.1	.302
20-24	1971.7	.266	1971.6	.245	1971.7	.261	1971.6	.999	1971.7	.261
25-29	1969.9	.239	1969.7	.232	1969.8	.238	1969.8	.236	1969.9	.237
30-34	1967.7	.231	1967.4	.231	1967.6	.234	1967.7	.227	1967.7	.229
35-39	1965.3	.226	1964.9	.229	1965.1	.231	1965.3	.218	1965.3	.223
40-44	1962.5	.227	1962.1	.237	1962.2	.242	1962.6	.218	1962.5	.224
45-49	1958.9	.232	1958.5	.238	1958.3	.248	1959.3	.210	1959.0	.226

NOTE: A q VALUE OF .999 DENOTES VALUE FROM TABLE WITH LIFE EXPECTANCY LESS THAN 35
 "   .000   "   GREATER THAN 75

Litho in United Nations, New York
89-40940—April 1990—4,075